1001 healthy eating miracles

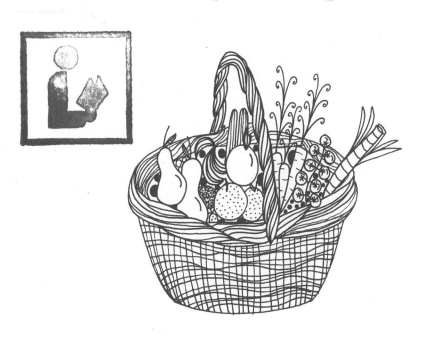

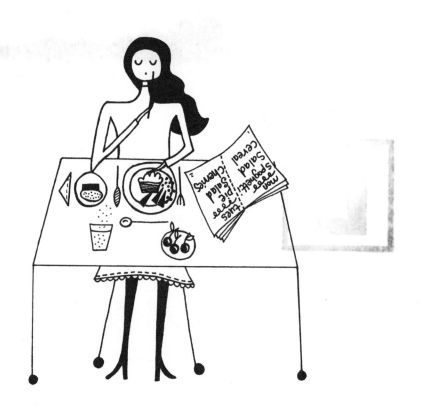

1001 healthy eating miracles

Esme Floyd

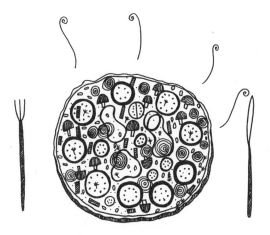

CARLTON
BOOKS

THIS IS A CARLTON BOOK

Text and design copyright © 2007
Carlton Books Limited
Illustrations copyright © 2007 Carol Morley

This edition published in 2007 by
Carlton Books Limited
20 Mortimer Street
London W1T 3JW

ISBN: 978 1 84442 068 1

Printed and bound in Dubai

Executive Editor: Lisa Dyer
Senior Art Editor: Anna Pow
Design: Ed Pickford
Copy Editor: Nicky Gyopari
Illustrator: Carol Morley
Production: Caroline Alberti

This book reports information and opinions which may
be of general interest to the reader. Neither the author
nor the publisher can accept responsibility for any
accident, injury or damage that results from using the
ideas, information or advice offered in this book.

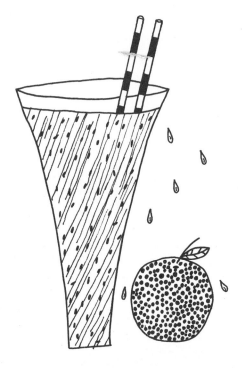

CONTENTS

INTRODUCTION

Did you know that you'll eat less if blindfolded, that ginger root stays fresh for longer if stored in alcohol, or that eating oysters could boost your fertility?

Here we've gathered together 1001 healthy eating gems to keep you happy and healthy in every area of your life. Packed with easy-to-follow tips, this little book cuts through the jargon to give you the facts about what and how to eat. Whether you want a natural remedy to beat stress, an easy way to drop calories or the lowdown on labelling, we'll show you the many simple ways you can make changes that will last a lifetime.

Top ten healthy eating miracles

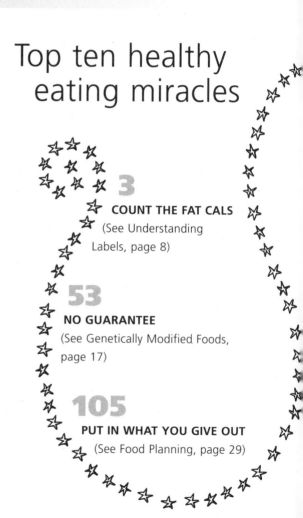

3
COUNT THE FAT CALS
(See Understanding Labels, page 8)

53
NO GUARANTEE
(See Genetically Modified Foods, page 17)

105
PUT IN WHAT YOU GIVE OUT
(See Food Planning, page 29)

271
MAKE A NATURAL CHOICE
(See Health Boosters,
page 67)

384
HAVE A GOOD EVENING
(See Ailments & Conditions,
page 90)

413
SMOOTH OPERATOR
(See Weight Maintenance, page 97)

553
AN EYE ON THE ALCOHOL
(See Eating Out, page 126)

610
DON'T DEPRIVE THEM
(See Family Food, page 137)

782
THE YOLK'S ON ME
(See Keeping Things Fresh,
page 177)

839
BE AN EARLY BIRD
(See Meal Planning,
page 189)

understanding labels

1 STARCH WATCH

The term 'modified starch' describes starch that has been physically or chemically treated for food product preparation, often for use as a thickener. It doesn't mean it has definitely been genetically modified. Check with the supplier to be sure.

2 JUST ONE DATE

You will see 'use by' dates on food that goes off quickly such as smoked fish or ready prepared salads, so don't use it after this date. 'Best before' dates are more about quality. When the date expires, the food might begin to lose its taste or texture.

3 COUNT THE FAT CALS

Make use of the 'calories from fat' label on your food. No more than 30% of your daily calories should be from fat – if you're eating 1500 calories a day, this is 500.

4 TRAFFIC LIGHT LABELS

Some supermarkets are adopting a labelling system of traffic lights. This signals whether nutrients we should be cutting down on – fats, sugars, salts and carbohydrates – are at high (red), medium (amber) or low (green) amounts per 100 g (4 oz) food, and enables the shopper to see at a glance if the item is relatively healthy or not.

5 FIBRE FILLER

Fibre not only helps keep your digestive system healthy but it can also reduce cholesterol levels. Best of all, it has no calories and it can help you feel full. Try to pick foods that have at least 3 g of fibre per serving, such as all-bran breakfast cereals.

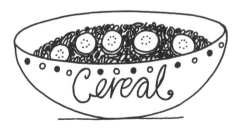

6 PORTION DISTORTION

Take note of how much a recommended serving is (100 g, 4 oz, 1 cup, and so on) and try to stick to that amount, only having more if you're still hungry afterwards. Often a serving size will be much less than you're used to eating – restaurant and take-away meals have super-sized over the years.

7 DON'T BE AVERAGE

Remember that recommended daily allowances are based on averages, so if a food claims to give 25% of the RDA of vitamin C, that's for someone consuming 2000 calories a day (depending on age, the daily average required by women). If you're consuming fewer than 2000 calories, one portion will give you more than 25%.

8 BACTERIAL BENEFITS

Check the sell-by dates on the yogurt tubs in the supermarket, and buy those that are most fresh. Yogurt lasts for about 10 days beyond the sell-by date, but the sooner you eat it the better in terms of reaping the maximum bacterial health benefits.

9 INTERNATIONAL DATES

When you're looking at use by and best before dates, be aware that different countries use different date formats. For instance, in the USA 07/03/07 means July 3, 2007 where as the same date in the EU/UK refers to 7 March, 2007.

10 GET YOUR DAILY ALLOWANCE

Each day your diet should balance out to give you 100% of your daily amounts for each nutrient. If a food has a daily value of 5% or less, it is considered to be low. Between 10% and 19% is a good source, and 20% or more is excellent. Choose your foods accordingly.

11 KNOW YOUR EGGS

Eggs labelled as 'Barn eggs' come from birds that live in a shed but are able to move around and often have access to perches, nest-boxes and litter, allowing them to forage and roost. These are not Free Range, which offers birds a similar interior to barn eggs, but also gives continuous access to open-air runs.

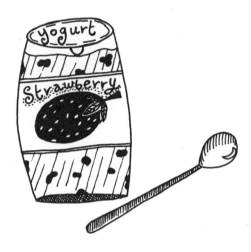

12 FORBIDDEN FRUIT

Choose foods labelled with the name of the fruit rather than 'fruit flavoured'. For example, strawberry yogurt must contain strawberries, but strawberry-flavoured yogurt probably doesn't contain any fruit and usually includes additives to create the flavour. Also, if there's an image of real strawberries on the packaging, the product's flavour must, by law, come wholly or mainly from strawberries

13 FOOD WITH FREEDOM

In the UK, the RSPCA has developed a farm and animal welfare labelling scheme that gives consumers the opportunity to purchase meat, poultry, eggs and dairy products from monitored farms. Look out for products labelled Freedom Food. Some campaigners say the scheme doesn't go far enough and it's still best to choose organic. Organisations in other countries, such as the ASPCA in the USA and the RSPCA in Canada and Australia, have similar food-monitoring systems.

14 SEEK OUT ORGANIC LABELS

The Soil Association in the UK has developed a certification scheme for foods that have been produced to their stringent organic guidelines. It is a recognized logo that, if it appears on a label, should reassure you that the food you're buying is as free of nasties as it can be. The equivalent in Australia is the Organic Federation of Australia, or in the USA choose food labelled USDA (United States Department of Agriculture) Organic.

15 GO VEGGIE

If you're looking for foods without animal products in them, look for those labelled 'vegetarian', which guarantees it contains no ingredients derived from animal sources.

16 CHECK YOUR FATS

'Cholesterol Free' or 'Low Cholesterol' means that the product does not contain any or only small amounts of animal fat or saturated fat, but it does not necessarily mean the product is low fat. Vegetable oils are cholesterol-free but made entirely of fat.

17 PLACE OF ORIGIN

Thirty per cent of consumers are concerned about country-of-origin food labels in the EU, which can be vague and misleading. For example, Welsh lamb can be sent to France, slaughtered there, and sold as French lamb – you would naturally assume that the lamb spent its entire life in France. Some labels read 'produce of the EU or South America' or 'produce of EU, Brazil or Thailand.' Ask the supermarket staff or your butcher to provide exact details as you have a right to know.

18 NOT THE WHOLE STORY

Remember that companies are not obliged to give detailed nutrition information about their food products unless they make a claim about their food, such as 'low fat' or 'high fibre'. In other words, something labelled '90% fat free' could contain 10% fat, which is a lot higher than the 3% it needs to be to be labelled 'low fat'. Check before you buy.

19 KEEP AN EYE ON SATURATES

Don't just look for total fat content on labels. The proportion of saturated fat – the really bad stuff – is important too. Products with 5 g of saturated fat per 100 g are classed as high-fat products, whereas those with 1 g are healthy low-fat options.

20 TOP UP YOUR FIBRE

Foods that are labelled 'more fibre' or 'added fibre' contain at least 2.5 g more fibre per serving than the original food, which means they are usually better choices. Do check labels, though, to make sure sugar, salt and fat haven't also been added.

21 SUGAR HIGHS

People with diabetes or who are worried about their blood sugar levels should avoid all food products where sugar is listed first under the ingredients' list and keep to a minimum products where sugar is listed in second place. These foods are likely to cause blood sugar peaks.

22 BEWARE OF HIDDEN SUGAR

If the label on your food says 'low cholesterol', what that means in practice is that it contains less than 20 mg of cholesterol and a maximum of 2 g saturated fat per serving. Be careful of hidden sugar in these products, which manufacturers use as an alternative to fat.

23 NON-LABELLED PRODUCTS

In the UK, shops are required to give basic nutritional information. For non-labelled items such as fresh breads and other bakery produce, check the price labels on the products in the supermarket – they should contain basic information and a list of ingredients to help you plan your diet.

24 PRESERVE YOUR HEALTH

Food which is labelled 'no preservatives' means exactly what it says, but don't confuse it with the label 'no preservatives added' – this is used to label food that could contain natural preservatives such as salt and essential oils.

25 A LIGHT TOUCH

Although some light products have certain guidelines to which they must adhere, sometimes the word refers to the taste or colour. For instance, 'light' olive oil has no fewer calories or less fat than regular olive oil – it simply tastes more delicate.

26 LEAN TOWARDS LEAN

A great way to get your protein without the added fat that often accompanies it is to choose food that is labelled 'lean', which means that per serving it contains 10 g or less of fat, of which 4.5 g or less are saturated, and less than 95 mg cholesterol. Remember that this is for an 85 g (3 oz) portion, though. Larger portions will contain more fat.

27 BE GLUTEN FREE

For coeliacs (those allergic to wheat) claims about gluten in foods are very important. However, manufacturers are not obliged to state how much

Gluten free

gluten is in a food item. As it is impossible to remove all the gluten from wheat, the gluten content may not be clear. Look carefully at the ingredients list to see how much the food contains, or choose one that carries the Food Standards Agency's Gluten-free label.

28 LOW-SALT IS BEST

Products high in salt contain 0.5 g of sodium (1.25 g of salt) per 100 g of produce, whereas those low in salt contain around 0.1 g, and medium is 0.2–0.4 g. Try to choose low-salt products whenever you can.

29 STAY BELOW THREE

Fat is usually measured in grams. A good rule of thumb for keeping to the right amount per day is to choose foods that have less than 3 g of fat for every 100 calories in a serving.

30 SEDUCED BY REDUCED

'Reduced' on a food label can be a little misleading. What it actually means is that the product contains 25% less of the specified ingredient (for instance, reduced fat or reduced sugar) than the usual product. Check the label to see exactly how much there is per serving.

31 SEARCH FOR THE SALT

Foods that are labelled as 'low sodium' or 'low salt' contain a maximum of 140 mg of salt per serving. This is a good label to look out for on foods that may contain hidden salt, such as soups and sauces.

32 THE LOW-DOWN ON SUGAR

In general, products are high in sugar if they contain 10 g of sugar per 100 g of the product. They are low in sugar if they contain 2 g per 100 g of product. Use this information on labels to help you choose. No added sugar means just that, and nothing more – it doesn't mean the product is necessarily low in sugar. Many foods (such as fruit) contain natural sugars, so no added sugar really means that no extra refined sugar has been added.

33 DON'T BE FOOLED

Foods labelled 'healthy' might not actually be terribly healthy. They have to have decreased fat, saturated fat, sodium, and cholesterol, as well as some added vitamins, but there isn't a specific amount by which they have to be reduced to carry this label. Check the label carefully.

34 WATCH OUT FOR PERCENTAGES

Beware of percentage labels on foods saying things like '20% more chicken' in a pie. This only means something if the product had a decent amount to start with. For example, if it's a 200 g pie that used to contain 20 g of chicken, that's only 4 g more meat, which isn't much at all.

35 FAT FREE, SUGAR HIGH?

Products labelled as 'fat free' or 'sugar free' are guaranteed to contain less than half a gram of fat or sugar per serving, but remember that usually products are only one or the other. Check that the reduced fat or sugar hasn't been replaced with a higher dose of the other to enhance taste.

36 CHECK THE LIST

If you're looking at ingredients lists, remember they are given in descending order, so the ingredient there is most of will be listed first and the one there is least of last. This is important in, for instance, products where you would expect meat to be the main ingredient.

37 SALT OR SODIUM

Some manufacturers make trying to work out salt in products difficult by giving sodium levels instead. Work it out yourself by multiplying the sodium content by 2.5 to get the salt content and try to keep salt below 1.25 g per 100 g.

38 BEHIND THE BIG SELL

Items labelled 'traditional' often contain a number of non-traditional ingredients, including E-numbers, and there's no law against using the word on foods. Check ingredients lists carefully to make sure it's not a marketing ploy. Other words that fall into this category are 'farmhouse', 'wholesome' and 'original'.

39 LARGE DOSE

If a food is labelled 'High in…', it will contain at least 20% of the recommended daily amount of that nutrient. Check the label carefully to find out exactly how much each serving provides.

40 A FRESH FEEL FOR EGGS

'Country-fresh' eggs, accompanied by a nice picture of hens running around in the sunshine, could come from caged battery-farmed hens that have never seen natural daylight. The same applies to eggs labelled 'farmhouse', 'farm fresh', 'selected' and 'traditional'. The only way you can be sure is to choose free range and/or organic.

41 LAY OFF THE JUICE

Fruit juice contains 100% pure fruit juice (although it may be made from concentrate), but a 'juice drink' only has to contain 5% pure fruit juice to get its name. That's a tiny dribble in every bottle and the remainder can be water, artificial sweeteners, sugar, colours, flavourings and even thickeners.

42 THE LIGHT TRAP

Versions of food that are labelled 'light' can contain up to two thirds of the amount of fat or calories of the usual version, so although they are good alternatives to fatty foods they're not necessarily healthy choices.

43 HIGH FIBRE FOR HEALTH

High-fibre foods are good healthy choices because they fill you up without adding extra calories. Foods that are labelled 'high fibre' must contain 5 or more grams of fibre per serving, so you know that if you choose them you're getting a really high dose.

44 FAIR DEAL

Buying Fairtrade doesn't just help local workers all over the world to get a better deal out of farming and producing foods. Because of the guidelines on how many chemicals are used to protect human health, it also means that fair-trade food usually contains far fewer toxins, too.

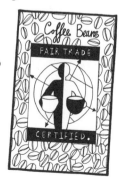

45 BEWARE TEMPTING OFFERS

You might be tempted to pick up foods that are labelled 'a good source of...' but beware – all this label means is that it provides at least 10% of the daily recommended value of a nutrient, which for some vitamins can be fairly small amounts.

46 SERVE YOU RIGHT

If you choose foods that are labelled 'calorie free', you can be sure that the food you're eating contains fewer than five calories per serving. Beware of serving size, though, as some manufacturers may specify small servings to get their product under the barrier.

47 LOW-CAL DOESN'T MEAN HEALTHY

If a food is labelled 'low calorie', it means there are less than 40 calories per serving. It doesn't, however, give any guidance on how healthy the ingredients are, how many additives it contains, or how processed the food is, so do have a look at the label.

genetically modified foods

48 HAVE YOUR SAY

Take a stand against GM foods by avoiding foods which contain GM ingredients and writing to the manufacturer to let them know about your decision. If only a small percentage of the population did this, it could lead to manufacturers losing sales and possible changes in policy.

49 CHOOSE ORGANIC

If you want to avoid GM foods, buy organic. Although there are a percentage of non-organic ingredients allowed in foods labelled organic, none of the ingredients are allowed to contain GM material.

50 MODIFY YOUR CHOICE

About 80% of processed foods contain maize or soya – or their derivatives – and so could potentially contain GM ingredients. Any label saying 'modified maize starch' or 'modified soya protein' is almost certainly GM.

51 HALF TRUTHS

There could be more genetic modification in your food than you think. Genetically modified bacteria and fungi are used in the production of enzymes, vitamins, food additives, flavourings and processing agents in thousands of foods as well as health supplements. Check with the manufacturer if you're unsure.

52 SWEETENING YOU UP

Aspartame, the diet sweetener, is a product of genetic engineering. By buying low-fat or 'diet' alternative drinks or foods, which may contain this substance, you could inadvertently be giving your support to genetic modification.

53 NO GUARANTEE

Did you know there is a threshold of 0.9% GM ingredients that foods can contain and still be labelled as GM free in Europe? This means that even foods that aren't labelled as GM could contain nearly 1% GM foods. Recognized organic foods, however, are guaranteed to contain none.

54 THE HONEY TRAP

The most difficult areas to control GM in foods are items like honey, where free-roaming bees may have visited GM-crop fields, inadvertently contaminating the honey. This is why Canadian honey is not on sale in Europe. Check labels carefully to be sure.

55 BUY ORGANIC DAIRY

Dairy products like milk, meat, cheese and eggs that come from animals fed on a GM diet do not have to be labelled as GM, so it is impossible to tell if the animals have been produced using GM or not. Buying organic will assure that they are GM free.

56 AVOID PROCESSED THE MOST-EST

The best way to make sure you avoid GM food is to avoid heavily processed foods, which are more likely to contain modified soya or crops. In fact, 75% of processed foods are thought to contain GM ingredients. The worst culprits are ready meals, followed by foods such as bread, biscuits, sausages, pies and chips.

57 BACK YOUR LOCAL

It can be difficult for those catering for high numbers – in schools, old people's homes and other mass-catering events – to be sure their food is GM free because of the large suppliers they have to use, but it's not impossible. Encouraging people to use locally sourced ingredients helps.

58 CORNY BUSINESS

In the western world, many crops are now routinely grown using GM seeds or processes. This includes 45% of corn and 54% of canola, which show up on ingredients lists as corn meal, corn syrup, dextrose, maltodextrin, fructose, citric acid, lactic acid and of course, corn oil.

59 THE BUTCHER'S BUSINESS

Many animals are now fed a GM diet. Visiting a local butcher will help you to remove these products from your diet because they work on a smaller basis than supermarkets and therefore should be able to tell you what diet the animals consumed, helping you avoid GM if you want to.

60 SOY SORRY

Most packaged foods contain soy in some form, which can show up on ingredients lists as soy flour, soy protein, soy lecithin and textured vegetable protein. A staggering 85% of these will be GM. Check the ingredients list, then scour the shelves for non-GM alternatives.

61 STAY OFF THE HORMONES

About 22% of cows in the USA are injected with genetically modified bovine growth hormone (rbGH), so if a dairy product is not labelled organic, non-GMO or hormone-free, it is likely that some of it came from cows injected with rbGH, which is thought in Europe and Canada (where it is banned) to have adverse effects on health.

62 LOG ON TO BE SURE

If you live in the USA and aren't sure about whether your usual food items contain GM ingredients, you can check them by logging on to www.truefoodnow.org, a site which offers an extensive list of foods by brand and category, indicating whether or not they contain GM ingredients.

63 GET POLITICAL

If you're worried about GM foods, it's a bit of a geographic lottery. In the USA, many foods contain GM ingredients whereas in Europe it's a much lower number. Visit your government's health advice pages to find out more about the area you live in.

64 CHECK YOUR OIL

Most generic vegetable oils and margarines used in restaurants and processed foods are made from soy, corn, canola or cottonseed — the four major GM crops in the USA. Unless these oils specifically say 'Non-GMO' or 'Organic' they are probably genetically modified. Non-GM substitutes to try include olive, sunflower, flaxseed and hemp oils.

65 WORDLY WISE

More than 50% of papaya (paw paw) from Hawaii is genetically modified to resist a virus so choose papayas grown in Brazil, Mexico, or the Caribbean, where there are currently no GM varieties.

66 THE FACTS

There is currently no real evidence that any GM crop or ingredient has a negative effect on human health or on the environment. But as there's no evidence to the contrary either, many pressure groups advocate avoiding GM until we can be sure.

67 LOOK OUT FOR HVP

Watch out for the ingredient 'hydrolyzed vegetable protein' (HVP) on ingredients lists, particularly for processed foods such as cakes, biscuits and other sweet snacks. This is a commonly used flavour enhancer, which is derived from corn and soy, so could therefore be GM.

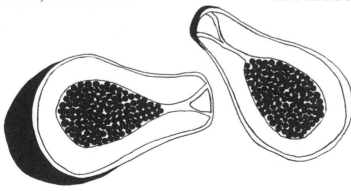

pesticides & chemicals

68 FISHY BUSINESS

In the past couple of years, the EU has significantly reduced the level of dyes that can be fed to farmed salmon because of concerns that the dyes, at high levels, can affect people's eyesight. If you have to eat farmed salmon, European will be safest.

69 FISH FOR PURITY

Oily fish show fairly high levels of pesticide and chemical residue. However, many of the fish tested are probably farmed and if you buy organic farmed or wild-caught versions, the residues are much lower.

70 REMEMBER TO WASH

In recent studies, the foods most contaminated with pesticides were found to be apples, peppers, celery, cherries and grapes. You should make sure you wash these items thoroughly, immersing them in water and drying carefully.

71 AND THE GOOD NEWS...

Not all food preservatives are bad news – the antioxidant food preservative BHT, which is used to prevent fat from going rancid in packaged foods, is currently being researched as a cure for cold sores. As with all preservatives, however, there are still so many gaps in the knowledge it's best to avoid them where possible.

72 CHEMICAL COCKTAIL

An astounding 447 chemicals are available to non-organic farmers, and around 31,000 tonnes are used every year. The most dangerous have been linked with a range of problems including cancer, decreasing male fertility, foetal abnormalities, chronic fatigue syndrome in children and Parkinson's disease, so choosing organic is safest.

73 WATER RETENTION

Chemicals such as pesticides and fertilizers sprayed on foods during the growing process are thought to be held for longer in watery fruit and vegetables such as cucumber and watermelons.

74 WHAT'S YOUR POISON?

Most people think fruit and vegetables are higher in pesticide residues than other foods but according to a report by the FDA in the USA, the highest residues are actually found in bread, flour and potatoes. Buying organic versions of these foods will dramatically reduce residues, although there may still be some traces.

75 ORGANIC IS BEST

While non-organic farmers have hundreds of pesticides at their disposal, only four substances are used on UK Soil Association organic farms – sulphur, soft soap, copper and rotenone. The latter two are 'restricted', which means that organic farmers must prove there is no alternative before they can be used.

76 A PLUM DEAL

The five fruits shown to be least contaminated with residues in the UK are star fruit, plums, peaches, kiwi fruit and hard-skinned exotic fruits like passion fruit and pomegranate.

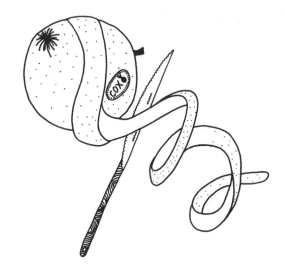

77 PEEL AWAY PESTICIDES

An apple a day is supposed to keep the doctor away, but the average eating apple – the most pesticide-heavy fruit – has been sprayed 18 times with many different chemicals. Most of the residues of chemical fertilizers and pesticides stay on the skin. If you buy non-organic apples, make sure you peel them or at least wash them thoroughly. This will also remove dirt and bacteria.

78 PILL POPPING

Total farm antibiotic use has increased by 11% in three years in the UK and many intensively reared farm animals in the UK are still given antibiotics in feed on a daily basis. The resistance built up by the animals' bacteria as a result is thought to contribute to antibiotic resistance in humans – and the only way to be sure you're not getting a dose is to eat organic.

79 CRACK THE CONSPIRACY

Many people think eggs are safe from pesticide residues and dangerous chemicals because they're covered with a hard shell, but in fact they are just as susceptible as poultry meat. Choosing organic will help you be sure your eggs are pure.

80 TRY TO RESIST

The USA has already banned enrofloxacin, a drug that causes resistance to the important medical antibiotic ciprofloxacin, which is added to the drinking water of chickens and turkeys. However, it's still in use in the UK on many non-organic farms.

81 BEST OF THE BUNCH

Among the foods found to be least contaminated with pesticide residues worldwide are asparagus, avocados, bananas and broccoli, so you can generally eat these without worrying, although it's still safest to wash before use. Other good choices are corn on the cob, cauliflower, marrow, squash and swede.

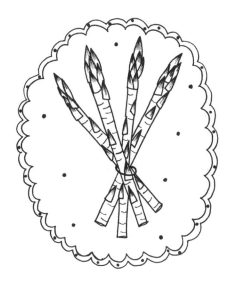

82 PICK YOUR PORK

The drug tylosin is routinely added to intensively farmed pig feed to control disease. It is also thought to increase levels of the hospital superbug VRE and to cause resistance to antibiotics used to treat food poisoning. Become an informed consumer.

83 LIVER YOUR TIMBERS

Be extra careful to choose organic when you're buying animal products where toxins may be concentrated, like offal. The chemical nicarbazin, which has been shown to cause birth defects and hormonal problems in animals, has been found in amounts up to 20 times the legal limit in chicken livers.

84 CAN YOU STOMACH IT?

In the past, the enzyme chymosin, used in hard cheeses, was taken from the stomach linings of calves. Since the GM variety was introduced in 1990, it is used in more than 70% of US cheeses. Its use is not allowed in organic cheese. In the UK, chymosin is used in the production of vegetarian cheeses, and does not require labelling.

85 WASH ORGANICS TOO

Don't assume that just because your foods are organic they'll be pesticide free. Most of the residues found in organic foods are probably the unavoidable results of environmental contamination in the past, or by drift when sprays are blown in from non-organic farms. Be sure to wash ALL fruit and vegetables.

nutritional guidelines

86 VARIETY IS KEY

Eat a variety of nutrient-rich foods. You need more than 40 different nutrients for good health, and no single food supplies them all. Your daily food selection should include wholegrain products (wholegrain cereals, brown rice, wholemeal bread, etc), fruits and vegetables, dairy products, and meat, poultry, fish and other protein foods.

87 BALANCE YOUR PLATE

Nutritionists used to suggest meals should
be one-third each of carbs, protein and
veg, but the most recent advice is that
your plate should be half full of vegetables,
a quarter carbs and a quarter protein.
Balance every meal for a healthy intake.

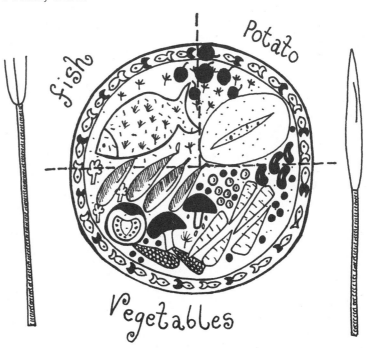

88 BULK UP ON PROTEIN

Meals containing higher levels of protein and a lower amount of carbohydrate keep you fuller for longer than those low in protein and high in carbohydrates. Alter the balance of foods on your plate to help maintain fullness, particulary at lunchtime.

89 AGE-RELATED ALTERATIONS

Remember that as you grow older, your calorie requirements will change even if you maintain the same levels of activity. Make time to think about your life-eating balance a few times a year to see if you need to alter your intake.

90 GROWING-UP DIETS

Teenagers and older children who are growing fast often have higher requirements for nutrients. For example 15 to 18-year-old boys need more thiamin (vitamin B1), niacin (vitamin B3), vitamin B6, calcium, phosphorus and iron than adult men. Similarly, 15 to 18-year-old girls need more niacin, calcium, phosphorus and magnesium than adult women.

91 CALORIE COUNT

For an adult man who is moderately active the daily guidelines are around 2500 a day. For women, who usually have less muscle bulk and therefore a lower metabolism, it's 2000 a day. Dropping 500 calories a day is a calorie-controlled diet.

92 SPOT THE DIFFERENCE

The main point of difference between US and EU/UK nutritional labels is that the EU/UK requires nutrients to be shown per 100 g or 100 ml. The nutrient amounts may, in addition, be given per quantified serving or portion (if the number of portions in a pack is stated on the packaging).

93 BOOST THEIR BRAINS

For children aged between four and six, growth has slowed down but general development is ongoing and rapid, so getting enough calories is really important. Studies have shown that children with healthy diets perform better in school, so aim to give boys of this age 1700 and girls 1500 calories a day.

94 GOLDEN OLDIES

Scientists have found that consuming a diet rich in wholegrain foods may lower the risk for cardiovascular disease and reduce the onset of metabolic syndrome, especially in older people so it's even more important to eat them as you age.

95 ALLOW FOR DIFFERENCES

Remember that US Recommended Daily Allowances (RDAs) differ from UK RDAs, therefore figures and statements of percentage contribution of nutrients could be misleading on imported products. Check where your products originated to be sure.

96 COUNT KIDS' CALORIES

Aged between seven and ten, children need around 2000 calories (for a boy) or 1800 calories (for a girl) to keep their bodies functioning optimally. Eleven to 14-year-old boys need an average of 2200 calories a day and girls a slightly lower 1900, but bear in mind that these amounts are calculated for average activity, so if your child is sporty, he or she will probably need more.

97 THUMBS UP TO CHEESE

Did you know that a portion size of cheese is just the size of a thumb? Or that one muffin or bagel portion is the size of a ping-pong ball? This means you're more than likely getting more than one portion with each serving, so take this into account when planning menus.

98 TODDLERS DON'T RUN ON EMPTY

If you have children aged one to three, try to make sure they get around 1200 calories a day from all the major food groups to meet their growth and energy needs. Try to keep down the amount of 'empty' calories – in processed foods – and to include as many different foods as possible.

99 TEEN SPIRIT

The recommended daily amount of calories for a teenager over 14 is actually around 300 calories a day higher than that for an adult because their body is using up lots of calories in growth and development. Aim for around 2800 calories for boys and 2200 for girls and avoid skipping meals

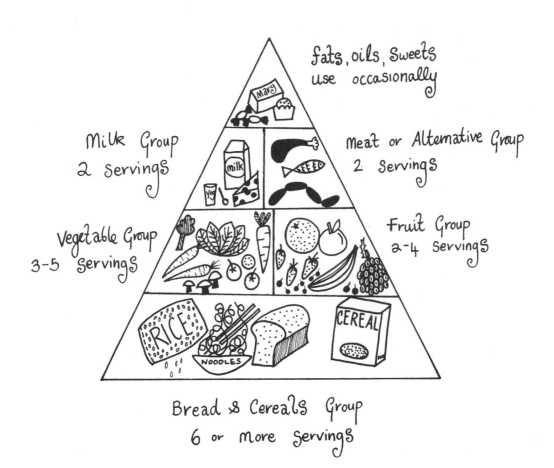

fats, oils, sweets
use occasionally

Milk Group
2 servings

Meat or Alternative Group
2 servings

Vegetable Group
3-5 servings

Fruit Group
2-4 servings

Bread & Cereals Group
6 or more servings

100 CLIMB THE FOOD PYRAMID

Many organizations use the food pyramid to help you understand how to eat better. At the base of the plan are plenty of breads, cereals, rice and pasta, vegetables and fruits. Add 2–3 servings a day from dairy and 2–3 servings from meat, and go easy on fats, oils and sweets, which are at the top of the pyramid.

101 DAY-TO-DAY NEEDS

Per day, the average 40-year-old woman should be eating 175 g (6 oz) of wholegrains, three handfuls of vegetables and two of fruit, 500 ml (18 fl oz) of milk or dairy products, and around 175 g (6 oz) of protein from meat, fish or beans.

102 EAT LESS EMPTIES

As a general rule, try and keep your intake of 'empty' calories (from sugary snacks, processed foods, alcohol, biscuits and cakes) to around 200–250 a day. These high-energy/low nutritional value foods should make up less than 10% of your total daily intake.

food planning

103 WEIGH UP THE WEEK

It's important to get a good balance of food every day, but it can be confusing and easy to lose track. To check, think about what you eat and drink over the course of a week – jot it down if it helps. If it balances out overall, even if you have the odd bad day, you're on the right track.

104 THREE OF YOUR FIVE A DAY

Most people know they should eat five portions of fruit and vegetables a day, but did you know that three of these, ideally, should be vegetables because they are lower in sugar and higher in fibre?

105 PUT IN WHAT YOU GIVE OUT

Start thinking about your balance of calories in and calories out. So, if you've had a really active day you might need a larger dose of carbohydrates to refuel your body's lost energy, but if you've been relatively inactive, you could probably make do with a smaller portion.

106 EAT ONE CARB PER MEAL

The best way to moderate your carbohydrate input is to limit it to one portion per meal. This would be equivalent to 1–2 slices of wholemeal bread, a cup of cereal, rice or oats, or a baked sweet or regular potato.

107 GO LIGHT ON THE CARBS

Watch the amount of starchy carbohydrates you're serving at each meal. Carb-heavy meals tend to be calorie-heavy meals. Don't be tempted to base an entire meal around noodles, rice or bread even though it's sometimes easier. Replace with more vegetables or a salad instead.

108 BE AN EARLY RISER

Get up five minutes earlier in the morning and use the time to sit down and plan your daily intake of food and drink. Knowing ahead of time what you're going to eat will make you less likely to binge and more likely to eat in moderation. If you're eating to weekly plans, use this morning time to revise your day's diet.

109 BAKE A CAKE

Instead of buying cakes or biscuits in the supermarket, make your own at home and substitute wholemeal flour for the usual white variety – it will make your homemade cakes nutritious as well as tasty.

110 FRUIT IN THE FRIDGE

Try fresh fruit salad for dessert instead of calorie-packed puddings. To make it easier, make a large bowl at the beginning of the week and keep it in your fridge so it's easy to dip into every night.

111 STICK TO A SERVING

It's difficult to know what's meant by 'one serving', especially if you're trying to count calories. Generally, the recommended serving of cooked meat is 85 g (3 oz), which is roughly the size of a pack of cards.

112 JUST SAY NO

Did you know that 500 ml (18 fl oz) of ice cream is the equivalent of four portions of your daily dairy and fat intake? Think about that next time you're offered an extra scoop.

113 TAKE A HANDFUL

How do you know what a serving of fruit or vegetables is? In general, it's about a handful of most types, or a medium apple, pear or orange. Bear in mind that for vegetables the amounts are measured cooked rather than raw. This is especially important for 'shrinking' foods like spinach.

114 SENSIBLY DOES IT

Always remember that effective weight-loss programmes should include healthy-eating plans that reduce calories but do not rule out specific foods or food groups, together with physical activity. This should give a slow and steady weight loss of 0.5–1.5 kg (1–3 lb) per week.

115 SERVE YOURSELF WELL

According to advice from the USDA (mypyramid.gov), for a balanced daily diet, you should aim for 6–11 servings from the bread, rice, cereal and pasta group (around 100 g or 4 oz), 3 of which should be whole grains. Then add 2–4 servings of fruit, 3–5 servings of vegetables and 1–2 of protein.

116 GROW YOUR OWN

If you're tired of not being able to find cheap organic vegetables, why not grow your own? Vegetable patches and allotments are becoming increasingly popular and they're a great way to ensure good quality produce. Tomatoes, lettuce and fresh herbs grow well on windowsills and window boxes too.

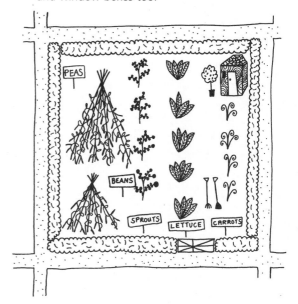

food groups

117 AN EVEN KEEL

Foods rich in soluble fibre have the ability to slow down the absorption of glucose into your bloodstream and to stabilize blood-sugar levels, helping prevent feelings of hunger. Choose oats, brown rice, barley, apples, pears, peas, strawberries, sweet potatoes, carrots and beans.

118 FEEL THE PULSE

For extra fibre smuggle lentils into soups and sauces. They are great if used as a thickening agent instead of flour, and give winter soups heartiness and flavour.

119 FAT BALANCE

Eat more 'good' fats than 'bad' (saturated) throughout the course of a week to get a balance. Good fats are the naturally occurring fats that haven't been damaged by high heat, refining, processing or other tampering such as 'partial hydrogenation'. The best of these are found in olive oil, oily fish, nuts, avocados and seeds.

120 EAT UP THE SKIN

If you want to give yourself a fibre boost, eat up the peel and skin of your fruit and vegetables rather than peeling and throwing it away. The skin is often the most fibrous part, especially in root vegetables. Wash or scrub them first to remove any lingering pesticides.

121 WATCH YOUR JUICE LEVELS

Although vegetable juice seems a really healthy choice, it isn't very high in fibre and actually contains quite high levels of sodium, which is the damaging element in salt. Choose low-sodium varieties if you can, and limit your intake to one portion (as stated on the pack) a day.

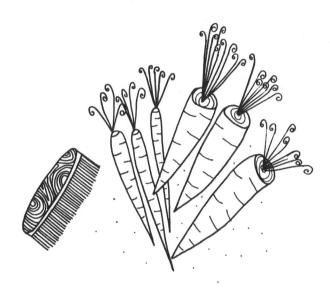

122 PUT ON THE PROTEIN

The addition of protein to a meal helps to slow down the absorption of carbohydrate into the bloodstream and makes you feel fuller, so you'll eat less. This means protein can help leave you feeling satisfied and productive for longer after eating, even if you've only eaten a small portion.

123 GET A FEEL FOR FIBRE

Insoluble fibre takes a longer time to chew and provides volume to food without adding lots of calories. It keeps your digestive system in good working order. Soluble fibre helps stabilize blood-sugar levels, warding off hunger cravings. There's some of both in fruit and vegetables.

124 BE PRO-PROTEIN

If you're a vegetarian, it's important to make sure you get enough protein – you should aim for 2–3 portions of milk or dairy products and two portions of other protein (such as nuts, tofu or fish) per day.

125 BEANS ARE BEST

Beans – particularly kidney beans, black beans and chickpeas – are great carbohydrate choices if you're trying to regulate blood sugar because they provide lots of fibre but are low in calories.

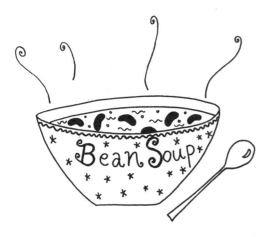

126 PROTEIN POWER

Recent studies have found that adding more protein (found in fish, meat, eggs and beans) to meals also has a 'thermic' effect on digesting your food, meaning it can increase your metabolism and help to burn off fat. Your body requires more energy (calories) to burn protein off than it does carbohydrates and fats.

127 DRINK FROM FOOD

Fruit and veg that have a higher water content – such as puréed vegetable soup and watery fruit like melon, celery and watermelon – can help fill you up, so you'll eat less throughout the day. Just drinking water does not have the same effect since it exits the stomach more rapidly.

128 PALM YOUR PROTEIN

The average woman needs approximately 85 g (3 oz) of protein per serving, and the average man needs just 25 g (1 oz) more (110 g or 4 oz). A serving should fit into the palm of your hand – a good way of measuring it if you're out and about.

129 MAX YOUR MONOS

Try to maximize your intake of monounsaturated fats (like olive oil, avocados, walnuts, almonds and sesame seeds) and omega-3 fatty acids (from cold water fish, hemp and flax seeds), which have health benefits for all the organs of the body, including the brain and heart.

130 EAT AWAY FAT

Put yourself together a fat-burning meal by combining green leafy vegetables with a lean protein source such as fish or turkey to form the bulk of the meal. Then add a small portion of natural starchy carbohydrates like oats, sweet potato, wholewheat pasta or brown rice.

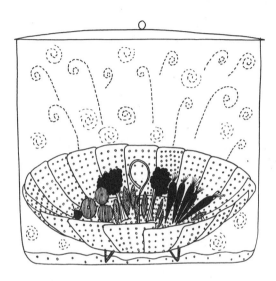

131 GO FOR GOOD FAT

Fats can be heavily disguised in foods, even with labelling systems, and it's often difficult to know how to get the right balance. To add good fat to your diet, cook with olive oil, add flax oil to a morning shake and try to include nuts, seeds or avocados in your meals.

132 FIGHT FATIGUE

Foods that combat tiredness include complex carbohydrates, potassium and magnesium-rich foods, and foods high in iron and vitamins B and C. Good meal choices to beat fatigue would therefore be meat or fish served with steamed vegetables and fresh fruits.

133 DON'T SEE RED

Try eating fish, chicken or turkey instead of red meat a few times a week. Red meat is a good constituent of a balanced diet, especially the leaner cuts, but in a healthy diet it's not necessary to eat it more than two or three times a week.

134 MAKE THE SWITCH

To help your heart stay healthy and give your digestive system a flush through, swap pulses or grains, which contain the same nutrients, for your usual meat or fish a couple of nights a week.

135 SATURATION POINT

Minimize your intake of saturated fats from red meat and full-fat dairy products, trans fatty acids from processed foods, and omega-6 fatty acids like safflower and sunflower oil, all of which can create problems in your body if eaten in excess.

136 BUILD MILKY BONES

Not only is skimmed milk lower in fat than semi-skimmed and whole milk, the bone-building calcium it contains is actually easier for your body to access because fat can interfere with calcium absorption.

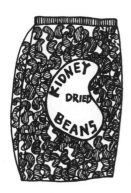
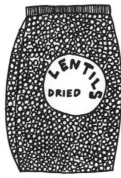
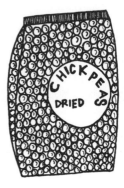

137 GET THE WHOLE PICTURE

To increase your fibre intake, which helps regulate the digestive system and boosts health, it's a great idea to include wholegrains in your diet. You can do this by using wholemeal pasta, oats and wholemeal flour in cooking.

138 KEEP FUEL LEVELS UP

Carbohydrates provide the body's preferred fuel: glucose. A diet rich in complex carbohydrates such as grains, cereals and starchy vegetables provides the best staying power because these foods are digested slowly and continue releasing energy for many hours after eating.

139 DRINK IN YOUR FIBRE

Soluble fibre is a really important part of any healthy diet because its soft texture helps your muscles to move food through the digestive system, for efficient digestion. It also boosts water absorption in the body. Drink water when you eat fibre for optimum nutritional benefits and avoid processed foods as they are low in fibre.

140 HALF AND HALF IT

If your family love the taste and lightness of white bread but you want to make sure they have their daily dose of healthy wholegrains, try using half wholemeal flour and half white flour in bread and other baked goods like muffins and pizza bases. You could also make sandwiches using one slice of white with one slice of brown, which looks attractive, is tastier and offers a healthy alternative to an all-white bread sandwich.

health-giving substances

141 HELP THEM TO GROW

For children and teenagers, it's important to ensure high levels of the amino acid L-arginine, which works with lysine and ornithine to stimulate the production of growth hormones and enhance infection-fighting antibodies. Good sources are nuts, sunflower seeds, chocolate, raisins and brown rice.

142 BE A GOOD EGG

Vegetarians who don't eat meat or fish should try to include eggs in their diet as a regular feature as these are the only other source of the amino acid L-Lysine, which has been shown to work with vitamin C to reduce damage to arteries.

143 TOP UP THE TYROSINE

Tyrosine is an amino acid that is a component of thyroid hormone, reported to aid in the treatment of depression, anxiety, fatigue and Parkinson's disease. It is found in meat, fish, eggs and dairy products and is better taken naturally because high-dosage supplementation has been linked to cancer development.

144 THE HARD TRUTH

Raw food is often richer in nutrients and enzymes and requires more chewing than cooked foods. This extra work is beneficial because it mixes the food with enzymes in the saliva to kick start the digestive process and ensure that you absorb as many nutrients as possible.

145 BRIGHT IS RIGHT

When choosing fruits and veggies, look for a bright hue – as a general rule, the brighter the colour, the more nutrients the food contains. Blueberries, kale and red peppers are especially full of antioxidants, which help to counteract the negative effects of pollution and the sun on our bodies.

146 SUP SOME SULPHUR

It's not only calcium and magnesium you need for healthy bones, skin, hair, nails and connective tissues in the body – sulphur is essential for the production of collagen. Find it in lean beef, dried beans, eggs, fish and cabbage, which are even more important to include in the diet as you age.

147 PRESSURE POINT

Vanadium is a required trace element that has been beneficial in treating some forms of high blood pressure and for reducing the body's production of cholesterol. It is also reported to reduce insulin requirements in type I diabetes, and is found in black pepper, mushrooms, shellfish and parsley.

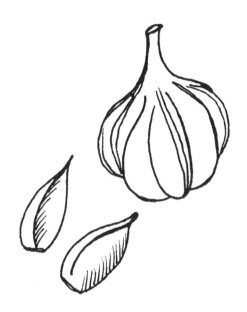

149 THUMBS UP TO FRY-UP

Next time you have a hangover, cook yourself a protein-rich meal such as bacon and eggs. It's high in the amino acid taurine, thought to help heart health and repair the brain, nervous system and skeletal muscles as well as improving the body's utilization of sugar and insulin.

150 MOP UP YOUR TOXINS

Foods high in sulphadryl groups are an important part of a healthy diet because these chemical compounds have been shown to mop up poisons and toxins, including metals like aluminium. Onions, garlic, chives, red pepper and egg yolks are all great sources.

148 DON'T BIN THE GARLIC

Don't worry if you're not sure whether to use that old head of garlic you've found at the back of the cupboard – aged garlic has been shown to have high levels of sallylmercaptocystein (SAMC), a sulphur compound that has been shown to slow the growth of prostate cancer cells. Fresh garlic doesn't have this effect.

151 CUT UP A CABBAGE

In order to protect yourself against cancers, it's important to increase your intake of plant phytochemicals, which contain tumour-busting enzymes. They are present in all fruit and vegetables but cabbage, broccoli, cauliflower, brussels sprouts and tomatoes contain the highest quantities.

152 MAKE AN ALPHA BET

Alpha carotene has been reported in some studies to be ten times more effective against cancer than the better-known beta carotene. Natural sources include carrots, squash, pumpkin, peaches, dried apricots and Swiss chard, which contain good amounts of both types of carotene.

153 ADAPT FOR HEALTH

To ensure you're as healthy as you can be, make sure your diet contains adequate levels of natural medicinal adaptogens such as garlic, echinacea, ginseng, liquorice, ginger, schisandra root and ginkgo biloba, which offer a health makeover in the way they adapt their beneficial qualities to individual needs.

154 BETTER CHOOSE BETA

Beta carotene is an essential substance in the body – it works with vitamin E against cancer, and with other vitamins against ageing and other damage, boosts immunity and promotes eye health. It's found in many foods but the best sources are broccoli, kale, cabbage, carrots, pumpkin, spinach, squash, sweet potatoes and apricots.

155 WHAT A HEADACHE

If you suffer from headaches a lot or your eyes feel sore and tired, make sure you're getting enough riboflavin, especially if you're taking hormone replacement drugs, which can deplete natural levels. Also known as vitamin B2, sources are milk, liver, yeast, cheese, fish, eggs and leafy greens, but alcohol reduces absorption.

156 GRAPE NEWS

If you want the benefits of red wine without the alcohol, drink a glass of red grape juice, which is also high in the antioxidant resveratrol and doesn't have the obvious negative effects of alcohol.

157 PEPPER YOUR DISHES

Why not use a sprinkling of cayenne pepper to help season your sauces? Derived from the plant *Capsicum annum*, it has been reported to improve circulation and to lower cholesterol. As it's a mild stimulant, it can also be added to hot water with lemon juice as an alternative to coffee.

158 THE RED LIGHT TO WINE

If you want to drink alcohol with your evening meal, choose red wine instead of white because it contains higher levels of the antioxidant resveratrol, which can offer protection against coronary heart disease. Try to stick to one unit a day for women and two for men.

159 THE RIGHT RATIOS

Omega-6 is added to foods during processing and is the main component of most low-quality oils. As a result, the average dietary omega-6 to omega-3 ratio is about 20:1, whereas it should be about 4:1. Getting this ratio right is an important step in preventing cancer through diet.

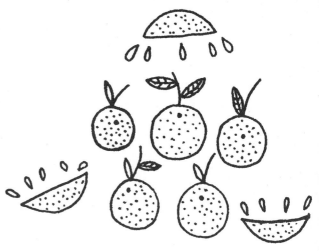

160 PICK THE PITH

Don't be too careful about peeling off the pith of your citrus fruits. Although the white flesh can taste bitter, leaving a bit attached to your citrus segments is a good idea because it contains high levels of bioflavonoids like rutin, which enhance vitamin C absorption and act as antioxidants. Bioflavonoids are also found in apples, blackberries and apricots.

161 BOOST CONCENTRATION

If you want to give yourself a pre-exam boost or sharpen your brain before an important meeting or presentation, get yourself a steak-and-egg sandwich which contains high levels of concentration-boosting choline. It can also assist in learning and help fight infection. Other foods high in this substance are beef liver, peanut butter and wheatgerm, or take a 2000 mg supplement 20 minutes before you need to perform.

162 THE SOURCE OF THE Q

If you suffer from high blood pressure, and particularly if you are taking cholesterol-lowering drugs which can deplete the body's natural stores, make sure your diet is high enough in Co-enzyme Q10 (CoQ10). Studies suggest it can help lower blood pressure as well as protect against heart disease, breast cancer and gum disease. Good sources include organic meat and eggs, rice bran, wheatgerm, peanuts, spinach, broccoli, mackerel and sardines.Try to include it in your diet every other day.

163 GEN UP ON GINSENG

Many people like to take a ginseng supplement, or drink ginseng tea, which has been reported to increase mental and physical performance. Vitamin C may hinder absorption, however, so don't take the tea with lemon juice and try to leave two hours between ingesting the two substances. Ginseng should be avoided by those with heart problems as it can interfere with the effectiveness of certain prescribed drugs.

164 GET YOUR QUINOA QUOTA

If you want to add a tasty source of low-fat protein to your diet, try quinoa, dubbed by some as a supergrain (although it's not a grass, and therefore not a true grain). It's high in fibre and other nutrients and has an extremely high protein content of 12–15%, making it especially useful for vegetarians. Quinoa has a mild, nutty flavour and must be soaked for a few hours before use to remove potentially toxic seed coatings. Use it in place of rice in cooked dishes or in salads or stuffing.

165 THE PERFECT PARTNERSHIP

The mineral selenium and plant-based chemical sulforaphane have been found to be 13 times more effective at fighting cancer when eaten together than apart. To reap the benefits of this partnership, combine selenium-rich nuts, poultry, fish and eggs with sulphoraphane-high broccoli, sprouts, cabbage, watercress and rocket.

minerals & vitamins

166 A STRAIGHT-A STUDENT

Excess vitamin A intake increases the risk of bone fractures and can cause poisoning of some internal organs, like the liver. For optimal bone mineral density vitamin A (retinol) intake should not exceed 2000 to 2800 IU per day. A good idea is to take less vitamin A and more carotenes (found in fruit and veg), which are precursors to vitamin A but have no negative effects if you take more than you need.

167 CUT BACK ON THE FIZZ

The body doesn't just need calcium to build strong teeth, skin, hair and bones – it also requires phosphorous. Keep the two minerals in balance for effectiveness (best sources are meat, dairy, fish, nuts and eggs). The recommended phosphorous dose is 1000 mg a day but too much is thought to prevent calcium being used properly. Fizzy drinks are high in phosphorous and don't contain calcium, so it's best avoid them if you want healthy bones.

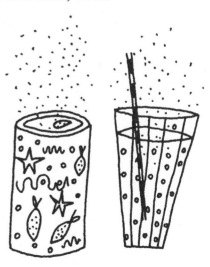

168 BECOME AN OYSTER EATER

Chromium is a trace element that the body
requires for sugar metabolism and
to control blood-sugar levels. It
also lowers LDL cholesterol,
triglycerides and body
fats. It is found in
high levels in oysters,
potatoes, brewer's
yeast and liver, and
the RDA is at least
200 mcg a day.

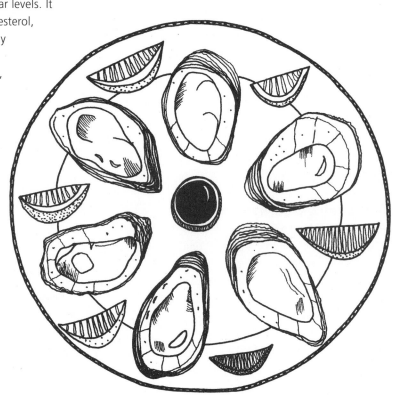

168 MEAT MATTERS

The best way to increase your intake of iron – particularly important in young women and those who have heavy periods – is to eat red meat. This is because the type of iron bound to muscle fibres in red meat is the most easily absorbed form.

170 BALANCE YOUR CALCIUM

Magnesium is used by the body in partnership with calcium to help lower cholesterol and build strong bones. In most calcium-containing foods, magnesium is present in the correct ratio (1:3), but if you're taking a calcium supplement take magnesium as well – roughly 500 mcg a day to balance 1500 mcg calcium.

171 GO SILLY FOR SILICON

The silicon content of the aorta, thymus and skin tends to decline with age so it's important to make sure you get enough of this mineral as you grow older. It will help prevent skin sagging and keep your hair, nails and bones healthy. Find it in grains such as oats, barley and rice.

172 PICK PICOLINATE

Zinc is essential for all-over health, including giving important protection against cancer, Alzheimer's disease and diabetes, but it is estimated that 90% of people's diets may not contain enough. Zinc picolinate is the most easily absorbed form, found in meat and shellfish. But caffeine, bran and dairy products can reduce absorption, so try to avoid eating them with your zinc sources.

173 BOOST VITAMINS WITH TEA

People who drink lots of coffee have lower levels of vitamin C and B vitamins and higher levels of homocysteine, a blood chemical linked to heart disease, than those who drink tea, which is thought to have some beneficial effects on the heart.

174 C THINGS CLEARLY

Humans are one of the few animals on earth unable to make their own vitamin C. Make sure your supply is topped up with a daily supplement for optimal nutrition, or opt for a diet rich in fruit and vegetables to boost your levels.

175 BUILDING BONES

Calcium, which is essential for building healthy bones, teeth and muscles, is best sourced from dairy products. Research suggests that dietary fat can reduce the amount of calcium absorbed by the body, so choosing low-fat or skimmed milk will help boost calcium as well as reduce cholesterol levels.

176 SEE YOURSELF RIGHT

Foods containing vitamin A, like melons, mangoes and watermelon, can help give your eyesight a boost as the vitamin is important for optimum vision. Try to include these in your diet every day.

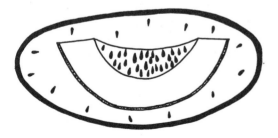

177 MISS OUT THE MARGE

Some studies have shown that people who eat margarine have a slightly increased risk of cancer compared to those who don't – perhaps because of the saturated fats it contains. A high intake of selenium and vitamins E and C, however, found in natural polyunsaturated oils such as canola, soy, safflower and flaxseed, is thought to offset this risk.

178 GET A BIT OF BETA

Betacarotene, which is found in dark green, yellow and orange vegetables such as squash, sweet potato, broccoli and greens, is converted in the body to vitamin A, which is vital for growth – so it's especially important for young people under 18.

179 SUMMER DANDY

Don't forget the humble dandelion when you're making up a healthy summer salad. High in many vitamins and minerals including the B-vitamin complex, it's a healthy and tasty way to make summer dishes a bit different.

180 BRAIN BOOSTER

Omega-3 fatty acids – found in fish, nuts, and flax and hempseed oils – are essential for maintaining good function in a range of body systems, including the brain. Nutritionists often recommend a supplement to keep levels up. A higher dose may be recommended for a few months to build up levels. No RDA has been established so check the manufacturer's recommendations.

181 BE GOOD TO YOURSELF

If your skin's feeling a little dry and jaded, give it an injection of vitamin E, which is an antioxidant vitamin essential for healthy skin, hair, nails and the immune system. Alcohol and lack of sleep deplete body levels, so if you've been out partying, try taking a supplement before bed.

182 DRINK IT FRESH

The vitamin-C content of fruit juices halves after a few days in the fridge, so if you're drinking juices at home, it's best to drink them as freshly squeezed as possible to make the most of the nutrients.

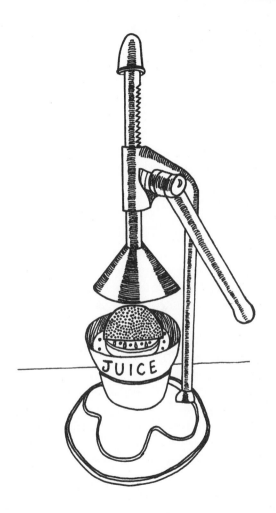

183 START WITH AN A

Adults should avoid taking more than 3000 mcg (µg) per day of vitamin A. Found in livers and food derived from them, such as pâté and fish liver oils, too much can cause health problems and you should be able to get all you need from your diet. Pregnant women should be extra careful.

184 BE A HEALTH NUT

Selenium is essential for preventing free radical damage in the body, and is available in a range of foods from grains to meat. It's just been discovered, however, that the body uses it best when it's in a selenoprotein form, found in nuts (especially Brazil nuts).

185 THE WHOLE STORY

When you drink orange juice, you get the vitamin C but not the beneficial fibre and phytonutrients that come from the pulp. Even if you buy orange juice with pulp, you're still not getting any of the fibrous white membrane, which is where many of the phytonutrients hide, so eat the pith too!

186 QUIT THE WEED

If you smoke, you probably won't be getting enough essential nutrients from your diet because tobacco decreases the absorption of many vitamins and minerals, including vitamin C, folate, magnesium and calcium. The best health advice is to give up, but if you can't it's worth taking a dietary supplement.

187 CUT BACK ON THE BOOZE

Drinking excessive amounts of alcohol can impair the body's ability to absorb vitamin B1, iron, zinc, magnesium and folate. Many people are surprised that excessive drinking is defined as more than two drinks a day for men under 65 and more than one drink a day for men over 65 and women. Aim for at least two alcohol-free days a week.

188 SPICE IT UP

It might sound old fashioned, but a pestle and mortar is actually thought to be a healthier way to prepare spices than a food processor. This is because crushing retains more nutrients than whizzing.

189 BERRY GOOD FOR YOU

Although tomatoes are the best dietary source of lycopene, there is an alternative if you don't like them – strawberries. These summer berries are the only other fruit or vegetable to protect against prostate cancer, and unlike tomatoes they are as potent raw as they are cooked.

190 COOK CONVENTIONAL

Think twice before you microwave your beef, pork, eggs, milk and cheese as you may well be reducing their health benefits. Microwave cooking (as well as alcohol, oral contraceptives and sleeping pills) is thought to destroy vitamin B12, which is essential for carbohydrate and fat metabolism.

191 SWIM OUT TO C

We all know the health benefits of vitamin C, labelled by some as the wonder vitamin for its far-reaching, positive effects on the body. People who smoke, drink alcohol or are taking aspirin, oestrogen or oral contraceptives should take more, as these can all limit uptake.

192 GO GREEN

Green tea is reported to contain a variety of antioxidants and to offer protection against cancer, heart disease and stroke. Black tea, which is oxidized green tea, is not as effective. If you don't like green, try oolong tea, which is only partially oxidized. But remember, all tea contains caffeine, so unlimited amounts aren't recommended.

193 SEEK OUT THE SYNERGY

Certain chemicals in the body work more powerfully when combined. This is thought to be the case for selenium and vitamin E, which have better antioxidant properties when present together. Selenium is destroyed by processing, so choosing unprocessed nuts and fish is essential.

194 WHERE'S YOUR BOTTLE

Tap water containing chlorine can soak up vitamin E and prevent its absorption in the body, so if you're taking a supplement or eating a healthy meal and your water is chlorinated, it's best to drink bottled or filtered water instead.

195 YOUR HEALTH IS OH-K

Don't forget about vitamin K, which is essential to maintain healthy bones and has been found to be lacking in people with osteoporosis. Antibiotics and the ageing process lower absorption, so in these cases it's even more important to get enough. Find it in green leafy vegetables, egg yolk and safflower oil.

196 SEEK OUT THE SUNSHINE

The body manufactures its own vitamin D as a result of being exposed to sunlight. People who work long hours and can't get fresh air every day might find a supplement beneficial, especially as lack of vitamin D is linked to immune deficiency and osteoporosis.

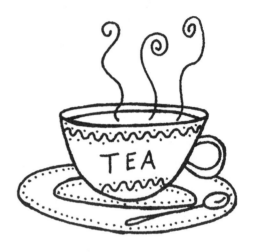

197 GET A HEALTHY U

As well as the well-known health-giving vitamins like vitamin C, there are a range of lesser-known substances which also have health benefits. Vitamin U is found in raw cabbage (used in coleslaw and salads) or cabbage juice, and is great for healing skin and membrane problems and ulcers.

198 HAVE A TEA PARTY

The caffeine in coffee is thought to deplete calcium levels, contributing to osteoporosis but the same isn't true for tea, which actually has the opposite effect. Drinking tea can reduce fracture risk by 10 to 20%, probably because of its oestrogen-building isoflavonoid chemicals.

199 BE A TART!

Choose tart fruits like plums, blueberries, cranberries and sour cherries, which contain the highest levels of the bio-flavonoid proanthocyanidin (also known as pycnogenol and adoxynol), which is thought to reduce cholesterol, prevent cancer and fight the signs of ageing on skin and internal organs.

supplements

200 A GRASS INJECTION

Superoxide dismutase is a potent anti-inflammatory and one of the most powerful antioxidants found in your body. Although it is present in certain foods, including cabbage, broccoli, wheat and barley grasses, it is difficult to boost levels through diet alone as it is broken down during the digestive process. However, a new type of supplement made from wheat grass has been shown to improve levels.

201 SWALLOW IT EARLY

If you take a daily vitamin supplement, take it with breakfast rather than later in the day, as studies have shown it to be better absorbed earlier in the day. And you should always take supplements with water, which helps absorption.

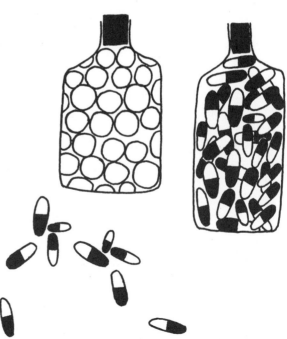

202 BONE UP ON BORON

Studies have shown immunity benefits and the prevention of autoimmune reactions (like eczema) in people who take 3 to 6 mg of boron per day. Boron also assists in calcium absorption, which maintains healthy bones, helps prevent osteoporosis and increases the synthesis of vitamin D.

203 READ THE LABELS

Vitamin C (ascorbic acid) is often made from corn, and vitamin E is usually made from soy. Both of these are heavily genetically modified crops, particularly in the USA, and vitamins A, B2, B6, and B12 may be derived from GM crops as well. Check your supplement and vitamin labels.

204 REMEMBER THE CARRIERS

Even if vitamins and mineral supplements aren't derived from GM sources, some of them – such as vitamins D and K – may have 'carriers' derived from GM corn, such as starch, glucose, and maltodextrin. In addition to finding these vitamins in supplements, they are sometimes used to fortify foods.

205 SWIM LIKE A SHARK

There aren't many stranger supplements than shark cartilage, but some people swear by it as an anti-cancer pill, inhibiting new blood vessel growth and stopping tumour spread. It has also been reported to reduce some arthritis pain, but it can be high in mercury so make sure your supplement is purified.

206 KEEP AN EYE ON THE IODINE

If you eat a healthy diet and are moderately active but don't seem to be able to shift excess weight, it's worth getting your thyroid checked – people who lack iodine or other nutrients could have an underactive gland, which leads to a slower metabolism. Taking 150 mcg of iodine a day could help.

207 PROTECT THE PROSTATE

Saw palmetto is a great supplement for men as it can help reduce some prostate problems, and for women because it has been linked with improvements in urinary tract infections. It is available as single supplements which can be taken as needed.

208 SUPPLEMENT YOUR TEENS

One of the most important times to give your child a vitamin supplement is during the teenage years when diets often become unhealthier. Choose one with vitamin A, riboflavin (vitamin B2), zinc, potassium, magnesium, calcium and iron, all of which have been shown to be lacking in teenagers' diets.

209 FOLIC ACID BLOOM

If you're pregnant or thinking about getting pregnant, make sure you take a daily supplement of folic acid (vitamin B9), which has been shown to help prevent neural tube defects in babies' brains. At least 400 mcg a day is recommended.

210 COLOURFUL CONNECTIONS

Eating lots of red and yellow onions, broccoli and squash is a good idea as it's important to get around 500 mg a day of quercetin, a bioflavonoid that can inhibit bowel cancer and protect against heart disease, cataracts and allergies. It may also have anti-inflammatory qualities.

211 GET PRO-HEALTH

Honey isn't the only bee product that's useful for keeping you healthy – propolis, a kind of resin produced by bees to protect honey stores, has anti-cancer, anti-oxidant effects as well as boosting immunity. Aim for at least 500 mg a day.

212 SUP SOME SEA HEALTH

If you just can't face the prospect of eating seaweed or plants harvested from the world's oceans, you can cheat the system by taking a supplement of phycotene. A natural extraction from spirulina algae, studies have shown it to support healthy eyes, to have anti-cancer properties and to protect the skin from sun damage.

213 BLOOD-THINNER WARNING

Not everyone benefits from taking omega-3 fish oil supplements – if you're taking blood thinners you should consult your doctor before taking these oils as they can also have a blood-thinning effect. In such cases it's probably best to get your dose from the whole fish instead.

herbs & infusions

214 DETOX WITH LEMON

Lemon juice is a great flavour enhancer and mixed with hot water is a really healthy (and detoxifying) alternative to heavily caffeinated hot drinks. Get twice as much juice out of your lemons by heating in the oven or hot water, or by rolling until slightly soft, before squeezing.

215 BREW YOUR OWN

Make yourself a herbal infusion from anise seed (*Pimpinella anisum*), a member of the parsley family that has a pleasant, liquorice-like flavour and is thought to improve digestion, freshen breath, calm flatulence and nausea, and help to settle coughs.

216 TUMMY TEA

If you are suffering digestive problems or diarrhoea, try blackberry tea. As well as a fruit tea, you can buy black tea infused with blackberries. The tea is rich in iron as well as easing stomach aches and diarrhoea and helping to control fevers.

217 TRY ALFALFA TEA FOR C

If you don't like citrus fruit but want to boost your vitamin-C intake, try alfalfa leaf (*Medicago sativa*), which is an excellent source of vitamin C a well as chlorophyll and other minerals when made into a refreshing tea or infusion.

218 PUT YOUR PEDAL TO THE NETTLE

Nettles often get a bad press because of their itchy stings, but cooking denatures the sting. Brewed up to make a tea or added to soups and stews, they are extremely rich in nutrients, including iron and beta-carotene, and are thought to improve kidney and adrenal function and help cure allergies.

219 RASPBERRY REPRODUCTION

Many pregnant women and those who are menstruating drink raspberry leaf tea, which is rich in nutrients, especially calcium, magnesium and iron, and is thought to help the regeneration of the reproductive system. But men can also benefit from its nutritious qualities, and often enjoy the tea-like flavour.

220 MAKE A MINT

A great post-dinner choice instead of caffeine-rich coffee is a peppermint herbal infusion. Peppermint reduces the more extreme movements of the digestive system, helping to relieve feelings of fullness, nausea and flatulence. It also has antiseptic properties.

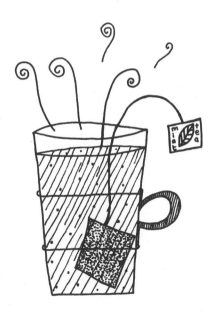

221 DRINK YOURSELF COOL

If you want the cooling, calming properties of a peppermint tea but don't like the slightly medicinal flavour, try spearmint instead. The flavour is milder but it still aids digestion, and also headaches, and has mild antiseptic properties. It also tastes great as an iced summer refresher.

222 TAME YOUR TANNINS

For the taste of a good strong cuppa but without the caffeine of normal black tea, try drinking Rooibos, or red bush, a traditional South African plant infusion that tastes much like black tea but contains no caffeine and is low in tannins and high in vitamin C, minerals and antioxidants.

223 MAKE A NEW MATE

A great alternative to caffeinated hot drinks is tea made from yerba mate, a member of the holly family, which is rich in vitamins C and B, calcium and iron, It also contains mateine, which is similar to caffeine but less likely to interfere with sleep, cause anxiety or be addictive.

224 WATER YOUR OATS

A great alternative to dairy products for calcium intake is water infused with oat straw (*Avena sativa*), the young stem of the oat plant. The infusion has a pleasant, sweet flavour, is high in calcium and is thought to relieve depression, insomnia, and stress. Try making up a batch and drinking it straight or using in cooking.

225 GET A FEEL FOR FENNEL

Try adding fennel to roasted vegetable dishes or salads – a member of the parsley family, fennel helps stabilize blood-sugar levels, thus curbing appetite. It also works to relax the muscles of the digestive system, reducing indigestion and wind pains.

226 INFUSE WITH FLOWERS

Instead of fizzy drinks and sugar-filled fruit squashes, try an infusion of elderflowers. These tiny flowers have a delicate taste, can be drunk hot or cold and have the added benefit of helping control body temperature – making them great as winter warmers or summer coolers.

227 COLD CURE

Many people recommend not drinking milk or eating dairy products if you have a cough or cold as it is thought to increase mucus production. A great alternative is tea made with lemon balm (*Melissa officinalis*), which has a calming, anti-anxiety effect as well as anti-viral properties – making it suitable for treating colds and flu in children as well as adults.

228 ZING WITH GINGER

A great herbal infusion to choose for an after-lunch energy boost, without caffeine, is ginger root (*Zingiber officinale*), a pungent herb that's not only good for digestion but also relieves nausea, improves circulation, warms the body, and has antiseptic and anti-inflammatory properties.

229 SIP A SUMMER COOLER

For a fantastically effective summer cooling drink, try an iced infusion of hibiscus flowers, which have a tart, slightly sour flavour and are rich in vitamin C as well as working to help the body cool itself when served cold.

230 CAMOMILE FOR CALM

Next time you're struggling to sleep, try brewing yourself a calming camomile infusion, which has been shown to have a mild sedative effect. Or if you want something with more flavour, catnip has also been shown to aid sleep.

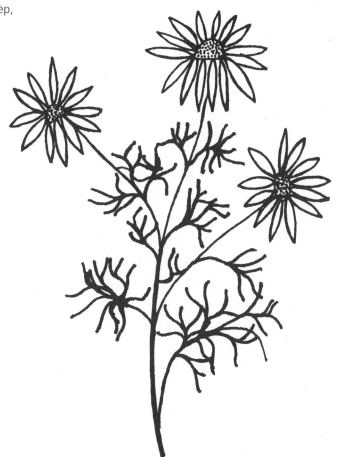

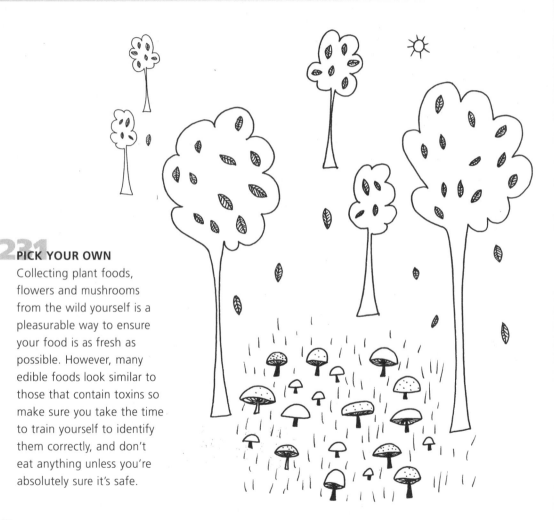

231 PICK YOUR OWN

Collecting plant foods, flowers and mushrooms from the wild yourself is a pleasurable way to ensure your food is as fresh as possible. However, many edible foods look similar to those that contain toxins so make sure you take the time to train yourself to identify them correctly, and don't eat anything unless you're absolutely sure it's safe.

232 COFFEE CHIC

If you can't live without the taste of coffee but want to cut down your caffeine intake, try an infusion of roasted chicory root instead. It has a delicious, coffee-like flavour without the addition of caffeine and helps to cleanse the liver and colon.

233 A WINTER LIFT

A great herbal tea to brew up if you're feeling a little depressed, especially in the darker winter months, is an infusion of St John's Wort. This plant is thought to help depression by stimulating the production of the 'happy' brain chemical serotonin. The standard way to make the infusion is to pour a cup of boiling water over the leaves and flowers, leave it to stand for 5 minutes, then strain and drink. See your doctor if you suffer from severe or long-term depression.

234 FIGHT OFF INFECTION

Help your body fight infection naturally by drinking tea made with the herb echinacea, eating the edible flowers or taking a supplement. The herb is thought to fight colds and to boost immunity by stimulating the production of lymphocytes, but it has not been proven.

235 GOOD PICKINGS

Don't eat flowers from florists, nurseries or garden centres or those picked from the side of roads. If they're not being sold for consumption, the flowers may be high in toxic pesticides and not labelled as is required for food crops. Stick to those properly identified and sold as foods – such as nasturtiums, dandelion and angelica. Always remember to use flowers sparingly in your recipes, as digestive complications can occur for those with sensitivities.

superfoods

236 GARLIC CRUSH

Garlic is great because it reduces the risk of stomach and colon cancer, helps lower blood cholesterol and reduces blood pressure. The ideal amount is 2–3 cloves a day. Crushed garlic has the strongest flavour, then chopped – roast is mildest.

237 A SAUCY TOMATO

Tomatoes contain high levels of lycopene and betacarotene and have been shown to reduce the incidence of prostate cancer in men if eaten ten times a week. The best way to get your dose is to eat a mix of cooked and raw to maximize nutrient absorption.

238 SPRINKLE SOME SEEDS

Seeds are packed with nutrients and beneficial oils and won't add too many calories to your diet. Sprinkle seeds on cereal salad, or, if you don't like their hard texture, grind a mixture of pumpkin, sunflower, sesame and linseed in a coffee grinder, and use whenever you can.

239 DON'T LOSE YOUR TEMPEH

For an alternative to tofu, try tempeh, which is made from fermented soya beans and has a meaty texture with a nutty taste. Tempeh contains all the essential amino acids and phytochemicals such as isoflavones and saponins, which are thought to help fight disease, as well as natural antimicrobial agents.

240 SEEDS OF HEALTH

If you can, choose ground flaxseeds over flax seed oil as although the oil contains just as many health-giving omega-3s, the ground seeds contain much more fibre, which is also good for health – giving you a double benefit for the price of one!

241 STICK WITH SALMON

Salmon is a great protein source because it contains fewer calories than many other protein sources, and it's rich in omega oils that help the development of the brain, heart, skin and joints. For the greatest health benefits, though, it's best to go for wild or organic versions.

242 EAT UP SOME SEA VEG

Sea vegetables such as arame and kelp are virtually fat-free, low calorie and one of the richest sources of minerals in the vegetable kingdom – they contain high amounts of calcium and phosphorous and are extremely high in magnesium, iron, iodine and sodium.

243 SIP AN ICED GREEN TEA

Home-made iced tea is a great summertime drink because it has flavour but no sugar and it contains antioxidants. Keep a jug in the fridge so you've got it on hand, or experiment with other herbal or black teas.

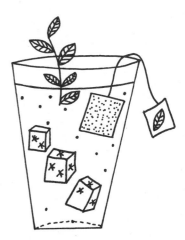

244 CLEANSE WITH SEAWEED

One of seaweed's most prominent health benefits is its ability to remove radioactive strontium and other heavy metals from our bodies. Whole brown seaweeds such as kelp contain alginic acid, which binds with toxins in the intestines (rendering them indigestible) and carries them out of the system. They are also sources of fibre.

245 CHOOSE NORI FOR TIREDNESS

Nori is a cultivated seaweed used to wrap sushi. It is exceptionally high in vitamin A and protein and a great source of selenium and iodine. It has anti-cancer effects and provides soluble fibre and omega-3 fats, as well as regulating the thyroid gland by balancing iodine levels.

246 TOMATOES SAUCED

Tomatoes are high in vitamin C and also betacarotene, which is converted into essential vitamin A in the body. They also have high levels of the antioxidant lycopene, which the body absorbs better when tomatoes are cooked.

247 CAST A SPELT

If you find wheat hard to digest and are worried about food intolerance, try replacing it with its ancient cousin, spelt. This tasty grain cooks in the same way as wheat but contains slightly more protein and is usually well tolerated by people with wheat allergies.

248 GET A GOLDEN PLATE

Try replacing your usual grain with amaranth, a tiny golden seed first cultivated by the Aztecs which is high in protein and calcium and an excellent source of iron. Amaranth is great as a hot cereal because it retains its crunchiness, or smuggled into baked goods or casseroles to add texture.

249 SPREADING GERMS

Sprinkling a couple of tablespoons of wheatgerm on top of cereals, casseroles or yogurts is a good health-giving habit to get into because it boosts the fibre content by nearly two grams but adds a paltry 54 calories. For a nuttier flavour, use toasted wheatgerm instead of plain.

250 GET A RYE DEAL

Did you know that barley and rye contain five times more fibre than other wholegrains? This is what makes wholegrain speciality breads such a great choice for your complex carbohydrate quota. Look for bread with these ingredients where you can.

251 SHARE A SHIITAKE

Shiitake mushrooms are thought to lower cholesterol, to stimulate the immune system and to help fight cancer. They are high in B vitamins and are low in calories so you can eat as many as you like.

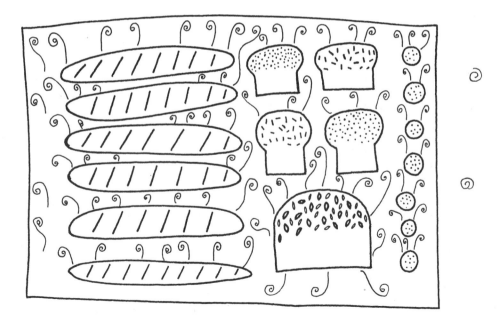

252 BUY BROCCOLI

Broccoli is one of the richest sources of antioxidants and vitamin C known, and the fresher the better. If you can't get it really fresh, choose frozen as it keeps its goodness for longer.

253 GET YOUR OATS

Oats are a genuine superfood because they have a low glycaemic index, which means they release sugar in the body slowly and help you to feel full for longer. They are low in cholesterol and high in fibre and protein. The easiest way to include oats in your diet is in breakfast porridge. For extra nutrients, top with dried fruit.

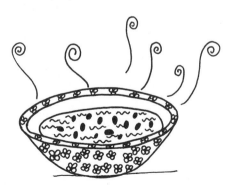

254 BE BERRY HEALTHY

Blueberries are a great source of the antioxidant anthocyanin, which improves blood circulation, skin and the immune system and has also been reported to improve balance, coordination and short-term memory.

255 BEANS MEANS HEALTH

For a great fill-up food that's good for your heart, releases energy slowly into your system to keep you fuller for longer, and is high in fibre but low in calories, choose beans. A recent study also suggests that eating beans and soy can cut the risk of lung cancer by as much as 46%. Experiment with the many varieties to find the ones you like.

256 GOBBLE A HEALTHY FEAST

Turkey is a great source of protein because it's very low in fat. It's also high in B vitamins, which help boost your body's health, and in the amino acid tryptophan, which aids restful sleep – making it a great late-night snack.

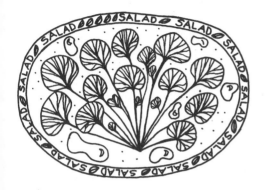

257 BE A WATER BABY

Watercress is being hailed as the new superfood because the chemical compounds it contains have been shown to help stop cancers developing by slowing down the degradation of cells. Use it in salads, sandwiches, soups and pasta.

258 TEA-OFF WITH CONFIDENCE

Next time you settle down with a nice cup of tea, relax in the knowledge that you're not only having a break but giving your body an antioxidant boost as well. Drinking it without milk is best, or with a slice of lemon to add extra flavour.

259 GO NUTS FOR GOOD FATS

Walnuts have lots of fibre and also contain high levels of polyunsaturated fats so although they are high in calories, the calories come from good fats which help balance cholesterol.

260 DO LIKE POPEYE

Eat spinach – it's rich in vitamin C, calcium and beta carotene, boosts folic acid and helps keep blood and bones healthy. Steam lightly and add to sauces or wash and use instead of lettuce in salads.

261 SWALLOW SOME SOY

If you're worried about cholesterol, add some soy to your diet. It's been shown in some tests to boost omega-3 fatty acids and strengthen the immune system as well as reducing cholesterol in the bloodstream.

262 A YOGURT BOOST

Live yogurts contain high levels of bone-boosting calcium and also probiotics, which improve balance in the digestive system. Low fat, natural yogurt is best.

263 PLUMP FOR PUMPKIN

Pumpkin has really high levels of potassium which can help control blood pressure problems, and it's also high in vitamin C and beta carotene, which both help keep the immune system strong.

health boosters

264 WARM IT UP

Your digestive system works best when food is at room temperature, so get in the habit of removing chilled food from the fridge a little while before you eat in order to let it warm up slightly. Food also tastes better if it's less chilled, so there's no excuse!

265 EAT LESS MORE OFTEN

Eating consistently throughout the day provides your brain and body with a constant source of fuel. This 3–4 hour eating strategy can dramatically prevent dips in your blood-sugar levels, something which is especially important in preventing premenstrual stress.

266 WATER IT DOWN

Drink water with your meals as well as throughout the day. As well as helping your body to absorb the nutrients from food, it also causes the fibre within food to swell, activating stretch receptors in the stomach lining to signal when you've eaten enough.

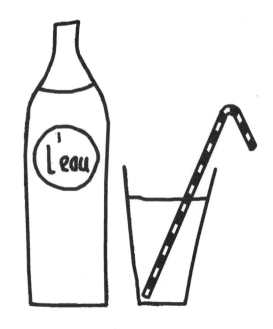

267 CHEW GUM

Chewing stimulates signals in the learning centre of the brain, which could help to preserve memory. Chewing gum also may, in a small way, help to keep you slim as it boosts the metabolic rate by about 20%. Choose sugar-free versions to prevent tooth decay and damage.

268 FEAST ON FLOWERS

Flowers are a great way to add colour to food as well as boosting health. For example, add the delicate blue flowers of borage to summer drinks to help boost brain function and immunity.

269 DON'T BE ACIDIC

Some scientist believe that for optimal health the body should be slightly more alkaline than acidic. For this, 70 to 80% of the food you eat should be alkaline-forming foods such as leafy greens, most fruits, soy products and seeds, and only 20 to 30% should be derived from acid-forming foods like grains, red meat and dairy products.

270 GO LIVE

For the best bacterial health kick, make sure the yogurt you buy contains live, active cultures and lists the Latin names of these beneficial bacteria. Many of the health-promoting properties of yogurt come from these bacteria.

271 MAKE A NATURAL CHOICE

Nutrition science research is finding increasingly that it is not one particular substance or another that gives foods their disease-fighting power, but the interaction of all the food's vitamins, antioxidants and other chemicals. To get the most benefit, try to eat food items in their natural form whenever possible.

272 FISH FOR VARIETY

When we're told to eat oily fish, salmon and mackerel immediately spring to mind, but don't forget there are plenty of other fish containing health-giving omega-3 oils in varying amounts. If you're bored with the usual suspects, try trout, sardine, tuna, pilchard, eels and herring.

273 REDUCE THE PROCESS

In general, the healthier choice is to eat foods as near to their natural state as possible. Choose organic and eat food raw, or lightly cooked. The fewer processes your food has been through, the better and generally tastier it is.

274 ALL RIGHT PETAL

A great way to add colour to salads is to sprinkle over some fresh nasturtium petals, which are high in vitamin C, or the seeds, which are high in iron and phosphorous. Both leaves and seeds – which are used in place of capers – are thought to help chest complaints and aid digestion.

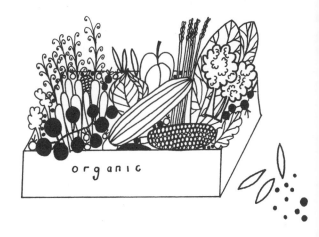

organic

275 CHOOSE CARBS FOR ENDURANCE

The body extracts energy more easily from carbohydrates, which it converts in to sugar, than from protein or fat, so if you have a really physical job or have an active day planned, it's best to eat a diet high in carbohydrates. Get them from vegetables, grains and legumes (peas and beans).

healthy habits

276 QUIT PROCESSED FOODS

A diet heavy in processed foods can lead to numerous problems. As well as the better-known obesity, cancer and heart disease, it causes rotten teeth, bad skin, bad breath, constipation, digestive problems, headaches, poor concentration, depression, tiredness and anaemia. Need any more impetus to give them up?

277 GO BACK TO THE ORIGINAL SOURCE

For each pre-packaged item of food you buy and serve, try to make it a rule to add at least one food from its original source. For instance, if you buy coleslaw from the supermarket, add your own fresh carrot, tomato or spring onions for a healthy boost. Or if you buy a ready-prepared pasta, serve it with a fresh spinach salad.

278 GET DRESSED

To avoid harmful processed fats, get in the habit of mixing your own healthy salad dressings. Try a mix of extra virgin olive or flaxseed oil, white wine or balsamic vinegar, and a little black pepper or mustard. Yogurt is a tasty alternative for creamy dressings.

279 VISIT THE GREAT PLAINS

If you have a daily chocolate addiction, choose dark chocolate as it contains less fat than milk chocolate and is higher in cocoa solids, which makes it richer and means you're likely to eat less. However, it does have double the caffeine of milk chocolate, at up to 50 mg a bar.

280 DIGESTION BEGINS IN THE MOUTH

Chew your food thoroughly – chewing, which breaks down the food into small chunks and mixes it with saliva, actually kick-starts the digestive process. In this way essential nutrients are extracted from the food and digestion is more effective.

281 CAN THE TUNA

In order to limit your mercury intake, which has been linked to brain damage in unborn babies and is thought to be toxic to adults, don't eat more than two tuna steaks or four medium-sized cans of tuna a week. Tuna, marlin and swordfish have been found to be high in mercury deposits and should be avoided by those who are intending to become pregnant.

282 BE A GRAZER

If you're looking for long-term energy, for shift work or prolonged exercise, for example, the best way to eat is to graze on small meals or snacks. This will keep blood-sugar levels up without having to divert too much energy to the gut for digestion.

reducing fat

283 SWAP HALF YOUR BUTTER

Instead of cooking with butter, choose oils that are low in saturated fat like sunflower and olive oils, which will help keep your cholesterol levels down at healthy levels and are lower in calories, too. If you want the taste of butter, try swapping half and see if you notice the difference.

284 IT'LL BE ALL WHITE

White fish is an excellent healthy food and although it isn't high in omega-3 oils, it is still a fantastic way to fill up on protein and essential minerals and amino acids without adding fat. Try halibut, skate, sea bass and plaice as well as the usual cod and haddock.

285 BET ON THE BUTTER

Don't automatically choose margarine instead of butter if you want to reduce calories – margarine doesn't actually have fewer calories than butter, unless it is specifically labelled as such. It simply has less saturated fat.

286 DON'T BE LILY LIVERED

Check the source of your omega-3 oils carefully. If possible, try to avoid those made from fish livers in favour of those extracted from the flesh of deep water fish. Pharmaceutical grade is the purest as it undergoes a variety of purification processes, so choose that for children or if you're pregnant.

287 HALF YOUR FAT INTAKE

All the different fats in foods can be confusing, but make your diet simple and give yourself a head start in the health stakes by aiming to make half of your fat intake polyunsaturated, and at least half of this oil containing omega-3s.

288 GET YOUR EGGS WHITE

It is the yellow yolk of the egg which contains the most calories, which explains the Hollywood trend for egg-white omelettes. In recipes containing lots of egg, try substituting two egg whites for one whole egg, or three whites for two whole eggs to cut calories.

289 LIMIT THE CHEESEBOARD

High meat and dairy product diets
generate excess methionine in the body,
which is converted into the blood factor
homocysteine that has been shown to
damage arteries and cause heart disease.
Reduce your intake of these foods or
increase your intake of vitamins B6,
B12 and folic acid, which help
restore the balance.

290 REPLACE WITH RICE

Reduce fat, increase fibre and save money by replacing half of the meat or poultry in a casserole recipe with brown rice, bulgur or cooked and pureéd dried beans or lentils.

291 OIL YOUR VEGETABLES

Instead of adding cholesterol-building butter to your steamed vegetables, make them even healthier by using a low-fat dressing or a dash of olive or flaxseed oil.

292 AVOID HYDROGENATES

Most UK supermarkets are starting to remove hydrogenated oils from some own-label ranges, but there's still a long way to go. These killer oils are even more harmful to health than saturated fats. Avoid them whenever you can.

293 CREAM OFF THE CREAM

Instead of using full (heavy) cream, which is high on calories and saturated fat, use evaporated skimmed milk instead, or low-fat yogurt. Or try mixing the two together for a slightly creamier texture.

294 CHOOSE OILS CAREFULLY

While most vegetable oils contain unsaturated fats and are therefore healthy, some – such as the coconut, palm and palm kernel oils found in many processed foods – contain high levels of saturated fats. Limit them in your diet, again, by avoiding processed foods.

295 TRANS-FORM YOUR EATING

Saturated fats are bad in excess but our bodies do need some for optimal health. Trans fatty acids (commonly called trans fats), however, are the real villains of the food world. Formed when vegetable oils harden and seen on labels as hydrogenated oils, they raise cholesterol and have been linked to heart disease.

296 ADD AN APPLE

Reduce the fat content of recipes by substituting half of the vegetable oil with apple sauce. You're unlikely to taste the difference and you'll not only be cutting the fat by half, but adding a dose of vitamins and antioxidants as well.

297 SWAP MEAT FOR FISH

If you pop to the sandwich bar at lunch-time, choose something healthy like smoked salmon instead of more fattening sausage, salami, ham or beef and you'll get a helping of omega-3 oils into the bargain.

reducing sugar

298 WHITE LIES

For a low-sugar option that's lower in calories replace white wine in recipes with apple or carrot juice, vegetable or chicken stock, with a little white wine vinegar or a dash of white grape juice.

299 TOP UP WITH FLOUR

Try decreasing the sugar in your recipes by a quarter, and substituting with flour to make up the volume. Most recipes won't taste any different and they'll be lower in calories. But don't reduce sugar in recipes containing yeast as it plays a part in helping the dough to rise.

300 SWEET ENOUGH

Look for unsweetened pure juices. Avoid products labelled as juice drink, which may contain as little as 5% juice and be sweetened with even more sugar than is found in a can of cola. Even pure unsweetened fruit juices contain natural fruit sugars which can cause tooth decay, but they are much healthier.

301 CUT OUT THE FIZZ

Unbelievably, despite all the media publicity about fizzy drinks being linked to skin problems, bad teeth, obesity and poor concentration due to their high sugar and additives content, they still account for 20% of the drinks bought for home consumption. Do your family a favour and make the switch to healthy alternatives now.

302 TASTE THE HONEY

Honey and syrup don't raise your blood-sugar level faster than fruits, vegetables or foods containing complex carbohydrates as long as they are eaten with a meal, where they are absorbed as part of the whole mix.

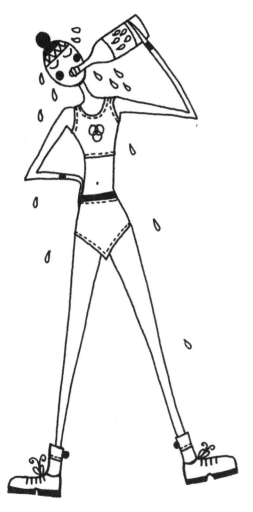

303 BE A SPORT

Don't be fooled by sport drinks, which are often marketed to appear as if they are a healthy choice but in actual fact usually contain as much sugar as other fizzy drinks. Isotonic drinks can be useful for refuelling after exercise, but water is a better choice throughout the day.

304 COUNT YOUR CARBS

If you're diabetic or are being careful to regulate your blood-sugar levels, remember it's total carbohydrate intake that counts rather than sugar. If you want a dessert, for instance, drop some of the carbohydrates from your main course to keep the balance.

305 SWEET-TOOTH ALTERNATIVE

If you simply can't cope with cutting out the sugar, artificial sweeteners like acesulfame potassium, aspartame, saccharin and sucralose offer the sweetness of sugar without the calories. They are especially handy as a sugar replacement in coffee and tea, on cereal or in baked goods – but it's healthier to go without.

306 CLOCK THE CALORIES

Artificial sweeteners don't necessarily offer a free pass for eating sweets, biscuits and cakes. Products made with artificial sweeteners still contain calories and carbohydrates that can affect your blood-sugar level and some may even contain sugar as well. Check the label.

307 TAKE CARE WITH SWEETENERS

Although sugar alcohols like isomalt, maltitol, mannitol, sorbitol and xylitol – which are often used to flavour chewing gum and puddings – are lower in calories than sugar, foods containing sugar alcohols still have calories. And take care because for some people, as little as 50 g of these substances can cause diarrhoea, gas and bloating.

308 DITCH THE WHITE BREAD

Swap white bread or pasta for wholegrain versions. Not only are they higher in fibre, they have a more beneficial effect on your blood-sugar level, releasing their energy slowly to help you feel fuller for longer.

309 DON'T BE FOOLED WITH BROWN

Most people believe brown sugar is a healthier option than white sugar but, in reality, the majority of brown sugar is simply refined white sugar with molasses added to change its colour. For healthier options, demerara and muscovado are good choices. Both are unrefined and suitable to add to hot drinks or for cooking, and have reasonably good shelf lives.

310 DILUTE YOUR JUICE

Instead of fruit squashes or cordials, which can often be loaded with sugar, dilute a little pure fruit juice with water instead. Fruit juice does contain sugar, but because it is natural fructose, the body doesn't suffer the same blood glucose peaks.

311 SPREAD AWAY SUGAR

Instead of jam, which can be packed with sugar, try no-sugar jam or make your own very healthy apple spread. Cook sliced sweet eating apples and a dash of cinnamon in a little water (it will keep for two months in an airtight container).

312 A SOUR TASTE

Along with refined sugar and white potatoes, overprocessed white bread is one of the worst foods for blood-sugar control. If you want white bread without the sugar rush, choose sourdough bread. It contains lactic acid, which slows down digestion and gives sourdough its tangy flavour.

313 LOWER YOUR SUGAR

To regulate blood-sugar levels the best vegetables to choose are fibrous varieties like broccoli, cauliflower, celery, cucumbers, tomatoes, spinach, peppers and courgettes (zucchini) and fruits such as raspberries, melon, papaya and cherries.

reducing salt

314 GO LOW-SO FOR HEALTH

If you like the taste of salt but don't want to damage your health by taking in too much sodium, try the low-sodium varieties – it's the sodium in salt that's thought to contribute to hypertension.

315 MAKE YOUR TABLE HEALTHY

High salt levels can affect blood pressure and heart health. Instead of using regular table salt in cooking, why not choose a low-sodium table salt, and leave the real salt for garnishing only? That way, you'll reduce the sodium in your diet to an absolute minimum.

316 CHANGE SALT HABIT

More than one teaspoon of salt a day has been shown to raise blood pressure, but for many people adding salt is a habit rather than a preference. Don't put salt on your food as a matter of course, and make sure you taste it before you sprinkle to see if the food really needs it.

317 BE A ROCK

Rather than buying standard table salt to add taste to dishes and on the table, choose rock salt instead. It has a distinctive salty flavour, which means you will use less of it, and gives all the taste with less of the damaging sodium. Plus, it contains 83 minerals and nutrients.

318 SWITCH TO PEPPER

Pepper is a healthier alternative to salt as a flavouring – it is said to aid digestion by stimulating the tastebuds and to reduce the formation of intestinal gas. It has antioxidant and antibacterial properties, too. Pepper loses its flavour quickly, which is why freshly ground is recommended.

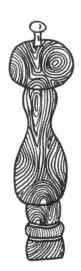

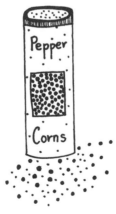

319 SALT AS YOU SERVE

Instead of adding salt when cooking, allow people to season their own plates when you serve the food. This will help cut down on the amount of salt in home-cooked food.

320 USE HERBS WISELY

Instead of seasoning with flavoured salt such as garlic, celery or onion salt, try using herb-only seasonings to reduce your sodium intake. Try garlic powder, finely chopped garlic or onion or celery seeds.

321 DON'T SALT YOUR SOUPS

Sodium from salt can be a contributor to high blood pressure, so make sure you choose low-sodium varieties when you can, particularly in 'hidden' salt products like soups, stock cubes and sauces.

322 SWEET AND HOT

If you eat a lot of stir-fried food, try substituting soy sauce, which is very high in salt, with sweet and sour sauce or hot mustard. Do this every other meal to help keep your sodium intake down.

323 CHOOSE UNSALTED NUTS

Nuts are a healthy, nutritious food but remember to choose unsalted varieties as salted versions can contain high levels of salt. Beware too of those coated with soy sauce or other salty products.

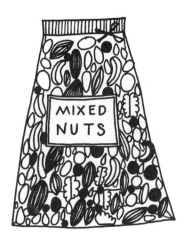

MIXED NUTS

alcohol advice

324 BEER WITH YOUR MEAL

Instead of wine with your meal, how about a glass of beer? Some studies have shown that drinking a small amount of beer with dinner helps reduce homocysteine, a blood factor that is thought to cause heart disease, by boosting the body's levels of vitamin B6 by 30%.

325 TAKE CARE OF YOUR HEART

Many studies suggest light to moderate drinking discourages heart disease, but this may not be true for men who already have it. Light drinking (less than half of the recommended maximum on an ongoing basis) was shown to cut the odds of death in men who did not have heart disease, but didn't show benefits in those who did.

326 RED REPLACEMENT

If you want the taste of red wine in your cooking but don't want to use alcohol, opt for grape juice, beef stock or water mixed with balsamic vinegar instead.

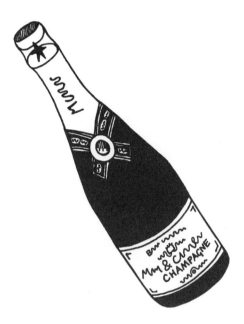

328 REDUCE THE SPIRIT

Next time a recipe calls for brandy, think about ways to reduce the alcohol in your food by using apple, white grape, peach or pear juice instead, or mixing half and half. You'll get the full, fruity taste without as many calories.

329 SAY BYE-BYE TO BEER

Instead of using beer to make a gravy for casseroles and stews, use beef or chicken stock. Stock will add flavour without boosting the calories as much as beer. For a kick, add a dash of Worcestershire sauce.

boosting fertility

330 PEAS IN THE BOD

For a nutrition boost which will aid fertility, add fresh or frozen cooked peas to your tuna salad and use spinach or watercress instead of lettuce as a base. As well as being low fat and high in protein, they contain the B vitamin folate, which is essential for reproductive health.

327 DON'T LOSE THE BUBBLES

Instead of champagne in dessert recipes, try sparkling grape juice instead, which has no alcohol and fewer calories than its more expensive relative. Or, for a stronger taste, ginger ale works well.

331 SPERM HEALTH

Men hoping to boost their fertility should eat more fruit and vegetables as a diet low in these fresh products has been linked to sluggish sperm. Any fruit or vegetable will help sperm health, and it's important to have five portions a day.

332 MORE THAN AN APHRODISIAC

There's some scientific proof that eating oysters can boost fertility because they are packed full of zinc, which plays a role in sperm production in men and ovulation and fertility in women. Aim for no more than the RDA of 9 mg a day as excessive amounts may actually reduce your fertility.

333 STEER CLEAR OF SOYA

A few studies suggest that women who are trying to conceive should avoid soya products because they contain a component that is similar to the female hormone oestrogen, which can affect the length of the menstrual cycle. Soya also lowers the levels of two hormones necessary for ovulation.

334 FIGHT THE PHYTATE

To maximize their fertility, men are advised to avoid soy because it contains phytate, which affects the absorption of the mineral zinc, essential for healthy sperm production. Another reason to limit the amount of soy consumed is that it is also thought to reduce the male sex drive – Buddhist monks have traditionally used it to lower libido!

335 EAT LEAN FOR SPERM

Lean meat in the diet releases ammonia as it is broken down by the digestive system, which can make the body slightly more alkaline. Sperm are well known to favour alkaline conditions, which means that eating meat a few times a week is a good choice to boost male fertility.

336 KEEP MEAT TO A MINIMUM

If you're a woman trying to conceive, meat can be helpful but it's best not to eat it more than two or three times a week. Too much can reduce blood flow to the uterus and prevent the egg from implanting successfully.

337 CHOOSE THE WHOLEGRAIN

Eating wholegrains is especially important if you have polycystic ovary syndrome (PCOS), a hormonal imbalance that increases insulin levels and can affect fertility. This is because wholegrains have been shown to reduce the symptoms of PCOS. Choose unrefined wholewheat breads with seeds for breakfast and sandwiches.

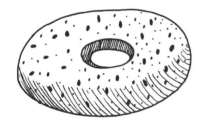

338 STAY OFF THE FIZZ

If you're trying to get pregnant, you should avoid diet fizzy drinks containing aspartame, which can affect fertility. Caffeine should also be limited as it constricts blood vessels, reducing blood flow to the uterus and preventing eggs from implanting.

339 DRINK ENOUGH

A high fluid intake is also important when trying to conceive. In order to stay hydrated, a woman trying to get pregnant should make absolutely sure she drinks at least 6 to 8 glasses of water and natural fruit juices (that do not contain added sugar) per 24 hours.

340 FISH FOR FERTILITY

Pregnant women should make sure they eat two portions of oily fish every week, or take a supplement containing omega-3 fish oils. Studies have shown that children whose mothers consumed these oils when they were pregnant perform better physically and mentally.

341 BOOST YOUR E DOSE

A powerful antioxidant, vitamin E is essential for fertility because it protects the egg from damage, which can lead to problems conceiving. It is also important in male fertility. Safflower, avocado, sunflower and wheatgerm contain high levels, or take a supplement to be sure.

342 CITRUS STIMULATES

Oranges and lemons are a good food choice for women who are trying to conceive because they contain folic acid, which stimulates the development of female sex hormones, while reducing the risk of spina bifida in infants. Drink freshly squeezed juice.

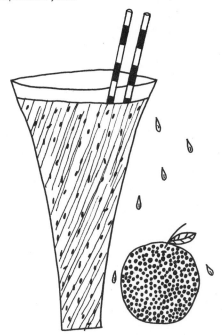

343 C THE DIFFERENCE

Increasing vitamin C to 500-1000 mg a day may help boost fertility in men by increasing the number and quality of sperm produced and reducing abnormalities. Get it naturally in fresh fruit or take a supplement daily.

344 CRESS THE RIGHT BUTTONS

Deficiencies of both vitamin B2 and folic acid have been linked with infertility, so women planning a pregnancy should ensure they eat plenty of foods rich in folic acid for at least three months before conception to build up levels. Cress and watercress are particularly good sources.

345 GIVE YOURSELF AN A GRADE

Vitamin A is essential for reproductive health as it maintains the health of the epithelial tissues that line all the external and internal surfaces of the body, including the linings of the vagina and uterus in women. Liver, egg, yolk, cheese, butter and carrots are good sources but stick to the RDA as too much vitamin A can cause health problems.

beating depression

346 EAT YOURSELF HAPPY

There are a number of foods that can help with depression. Eating a high carbohydrate (wholewheat) diet boosts the production of serotonin in the brain, making you feel more positive. Eating plenty of protein to increase amino acid intake has the same effect.

347 B-EAT DEPRESSION

B vitamins, especially B12, B6 and folic acid, can help combat psychological disturbances, so if you're suffering from depression a complete vitamin and mineral supplement containing these substances might help.

348 OIL AWAY WORRIES

Omega-3 has been shown to help depression by altering the way the brain functions and reducing negative thoughts. It is not known exactly how this works, but some scientists believe it makes the uptake of brain chemicals such as serotonin more efficient.

349 GO LOW-GI

Too many fluctuations in your insulin levels can lead to mood swings and fatigue, and these will be much worse if you already suffer from depression. To combat these ups and downs eat carbohydrates with a low glycaemic index such as basmati rice, couscous, oats or bran.

350 CONCENTRATE ON CARBS

People who suffer depression should steer clear of low-carb diets, even if they want to lose weight. Instead, eat wholegrain carbohydrates and swap unhealthy foods for salmon and mackerel, spinach, fresh peas, chickpeas, chicken and turkey.

351 SCOOP A GOOD MOOD

It's official – children have known it for years, but scientists now admit that eating ice cream can actually make you feel better. Eating a spoonful of ice cream lights up the same pleasure centre in the brain as winning money. Unfortunately, eating more doesn't give more pleasure and, as it's high in fat, one spoonful is enough!

352 CANOLA CAN HELP

Some studies have' shown that people who suffer from depression also have lower levels of the antioxidant vitamin E. Canola oil is rich in vitamin E so try substituting it for vegetable oil in cooking.

353 BOOST MOOD WITH FOLATE

Folate (also known as folic acid or vitamin B9) – found in many vegetables but most readily in the dark green, leafy varieties – is essential for the production of serotonin in the brain, which helps to regulate mood. Get happy with broccoli, spinach, kale and watercress. Some breakfast cereals are also fortified with folate/folic acid – Check the label.

354 GET REGULAR

Vitamin B6 plays an essential role in regulating brain chemicals, particularly when it comes to ensuring serotonin levels are high enough. Chicken and turkey are great sources of B6, which means they're good food choices to help regulate moods.

pregnancy & menopause

355 ALL FOR ALFALFA

Alfalfa sprouts are rich in phytoestrogens, especially isoflavones, which help relieve menopausal symptoms, as well as osteoporosis, cancer and heart disease, while cress is high in folic acid. Add sprouts to your salads and sandwich fillings for all-round women's health.

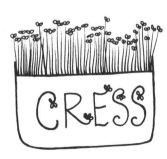

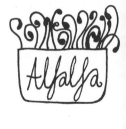

356 SMALL FRY

If you're worried about mercury levels in fish and want to eat oil fish, choose those lowest down the food chain, where the toxic metal hasn't had a chance to accumulate. Sardines, mackerel, anchovies and pilchards are good choices.

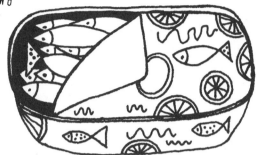

357 TAINTED WITH TOXINS

Mercury is toxic to an unborn foetus and can stay in the bloodstream for over a year. Fish high in mercury include shark, swordfish and marlin. Fish that contain low levels include salmon, flounder, trout, haddock, tilapia and yellow fin tuna so choose these to be safe if you're pregnant or trying to conceive.

358 SUP A SUPPLEMENT

After menopause, women experience a sudden drop in oestrogen levels which increases bone loss. To keep bones strong you need calcium and also vitamin D, which helps the body use calcium. If your diet isn't rich in these substances, a vitamin supplement is a good idea.

359 BREAST-FEEDING EXTRA

Remember that if you're breastfeeding you'll need to consume an extra 300 calories a day to ensure your child gets the most benefit from your breast milk. This is the equivalent of a piece of wholemeal toast with butter, a full fat yogurt and a banana.

360 FLAX FACTS

Many pregnant women and vegetarians feel wary about eating fish but may be concerned they're not getting enough omega-3 fats. For these women, flax seeds are another good source, and extra omega-3 is now being added to many foods, including yogurts and breads.

361 DROP NUTS FOR YOUR BABY

If you're pregnant, it's worth avoiding nuts, particularly peanuts, if the baby is at risk of developing allergies. Avoid them if you or the baby's father, brothers or sisters have certain allergic conditions such as hayfever, asthma and/or eczema.

362 IRON OUT PROBLEMS

Low iron levels at the onset of pregnancy increase the risk of developing anaemia after the baby is born. This affects almost a third of women, reducing energy. It can also contribute to postnatal depression. To maintain good iron levels eat lean red meat, fortified breakfast cereals, eggs, pulses, green leafy vegetables, dried apricots and prunes and wholegrain bread.

363 GRATE SOME GINGER

A great way to stave off nausea caused by pregnancy or other illness is to make yourself an infusion of ginger and lemon juice – not only will it calm your stomach, it will give you a vitamin boost too. Fresh ginger is the most beneficial.

364 HAPPY GRAZING

If you're pregnant or thinking of trying to conceive, it's important to snack regularly if you're hungry – pregnancy isn't the time to watch your weight. Women with regulated blood sugar levels (ie, who didn't let themselves get hungry) are thought to have children who perform better in brain function and memory.

365 KEEP UP THE CALCIUM

Pregnant women should aim for at least 1000 mg of calcium a day, which is more than women who aren't pregnant. Dairy products are a great source, avoiding those that are made with mould, and there is also calcium in meat and fish and green vegetables. Low-fat yogurts, cottage cheese and dried apricots make good snacks.

366 CAFFEINE CONSCIOUS

Pregnant women should limit their intake of caffeine as more 300 mg per day (three cups of coffee, 6 cups of tea or 8 cans of cola) has been linked to miscarriage and low birth weight.

ailments & conditions

367 REDUCE INFLAMMATION

Not only is oily fish great for brain function and skin and organ health, it's also likely to be beneficial if you have an inflammatory type of arthritis (such as rheumatoid, reactive or psoriatic arthritis, or ankylosing spondylitis), as it contains anti-inflammatory essential fatty acids.

368 EAT TO SLEEP

If you have sleep problems, choosing the right foods and drinks in the evening might help. Steer clear of high-GI foods that boost energy and caffeine drinks, opting instead for foods containing the amino acid tryptophan such as lettuce, brown bread and turkey.

369 PROTECT YOUR GUMS

Not only is gum disease unattractive and painful, it has also been linked with other more serious problems like strokes and heart disease. Eating a diet as low in refined sugars as possible helps.

370 SO SOYA FOR THE LACTOSE INTOLERANT

Soy milk is an ideal alternative to cow's milk for those who suffer from an intolerance to lactose. Soy protein has also been found to actively lower cholesterol and help to maintain a healthy heart. Substitute soya milk for cow's milk in your daily latte and reap the benefits.

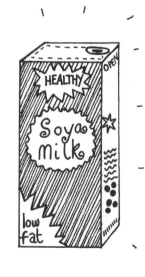

371 SLEEP LIKE A BABY

For a healthy, sleep-inducing midnight snack choose foods high in melatonin, which is said to protect against cancer and the damage caused by ageing and the sun, and has been shown to be good at treating insomnia. Try sweetcorn, rice, ginger, tomatoes, bananas and barley.

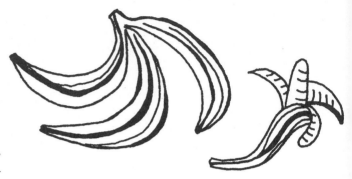

372 CUT THE ACIDS

There is no scientific evidence to prove 'arthritis diets' work, but many sufferers swear by cutting out acidic fruit and solanaceous plants like potatoes, tomatoes, peppers and aubergines, or by adding honey and cider vinegar to their diet.

373 EAT FOR YOUR EYES

It isn't only good for your heart and brain – eating fish can also protect your eyes from age-related macular degeneration, a potential cause of blindness. People who eat fish more than once a week are only half as likely to develop the disease as those who don't.

374 OIL YOUR JOINTS

We all know that fish oils help fight arthritis, but olive oil can also help protect against this inflammatory disease. It is said that those who eat it every day reduce their risk by 2.5 times, possibly because of its high levels of antioxidants.

375 FIGHT FUNGUS WITH LINSEED

Health problems which are due to yeast or fungus overloads in the body – like thrush or athlete's foot – can be reduced by taking a few teaspoons of linseed oil once or twice a day, as directed.

376 GO FOR GARLIC

Adding garlic to sauces is a great health booster because it contains high levels of germanium and allium, thought to have anti-inflammatory, anti-viral and tumour fighting properties, as well as fighting arthritis. Some people choose deodorized garlic, but the smelly kind has more health benefits.

377 TURN OFF THE TAP

People who drink too much tap water (more than the daily recommended dose) have been shown in some countries to have an increased chance of developing bladder cancer than those who drank other forms. Tap water contains chlorine, which has been linked to cancers, and the toxin arsenic, which has been linked to bladder cancer.

378 CUT THE COFFEE

People who drink three cups of coffee or less each day are half as likely to develop rheumatoid arthritis as those who drink four or more, and oils in unfiltered coffee can raise cholesterol levels. Cut down coffee intake or switch to decaf to be sure.

379 PROTECT YOUR BREASTS

Milk doesn't only contribute to health by adding calcium and – if low-fat versions are drunk – reducing the body's absorption of fat, it has also been shown to reduce breast cancer risk by almost half in women who drink the equivalent of three glasses a day.

380 KEEP SUGAR LOW

The body needs some sugar in the diet, so it's best not to cut it out completely, but high levels of sugar, especially snacks between meals, which lead to dramatic insulin peaks, have been linked with breast cancer and colon cancer as well as cholesterol levels. Cutting down is best.

381 GRAPEFRUIT WARNING

The juice of grapefruits has chemicals in it which have been shown to cause harmful side effects if taken with certain medicines. If you are taking medications on a regular basis, and if you want to drink grapefruit juice or eat grapefruit regularly, check with your doctor or pharmacist to see if you are at risk.

382 CURRYING FLAVOUR

Sprinkling meals with turmeric is a good idea because the herb has been reported to prevent blood clots, reduce the pain and inflammation associated with arthritis and lower cholesterol. It's good on spicy foods and with vegetables.

383 CRAM IN THE CRANBERRY

A couple of glasses of cranberry juice a day can help prevent urinary tract infections, especially in older women, by preventing bacteria from sticking to the walls of the bladder. It can also help prevent cystitis in younger women. Buy the highest concentrate you can find.

384 HAVE A GOOD EVENING

Evening primrose oil contains around 9% omega-6 fatty acids, which are needed by the body for hormone production and to reduce inflammation. This wonder oil is also credited with reducing blood pressure, helping fight depression and reducing the symptoms of PMS.

385 SMOOTH OUT JOINT PROBLEMS

One of the best food supplements for healthy joints, especially in older people, is glucosamine sulphate, which has been shown to help the body replenish the cartilage in joints, reducing joint pain dramatically if 1000 mg is taken daily.

386 FIGHT FATIGUE

If you spend a lot of time feeling tired, or you have whole days where you just can't seem to wake up, think about reducing your caffeine and sugar intake. They both drain your adrenals, whose job it is to regulate energy. It is easier to cut down a little at a time rather than going cold turkey, which can lead to headaches.

387 REDUCE STRESS WITH FISH

Eating oily fish has been shown to reduce stress hormones by almost a quarter as well as boosting anti-stress hormones in the body – making it the perfect choice for a working lunch to set you up for a productive afternoon.

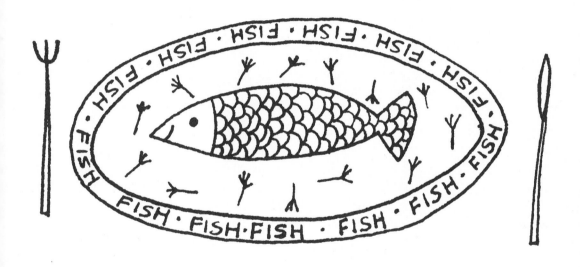

weight maintenance

388 TAKE AN EVENING OFF

Even people who are dieting can have a night off once in a while! Decide what you're going to have and allow yourself to indulge for the evening, but make it one night only – it's back to healthy eating the next day!

389 WATER FILLER

Your body can often confuse hunger with thirst, so next time you think you're hungry try first drinking a glass of water before you reach for the snacks. That way, you'll start to read your body's signs better and only snack when you're genuinely hungry.

390 DON'T SKIP TO BE SLIM

Many people think skipping a meal makes it easier to cut calories, but you will actually be more likely to overeat later. Instead, aim to have three balanced meals per day plus two or three small healthy snacks.

391 DOUBLE UP ON WEIGHT LOSS

Take a two-pronged approach to losing weight to make it sustainable – instead of trying to cut, say, 500 calories a day from your diet, cut out half the amount and make up the rest with exercise. This would mean cutting out 250 calories and burning off a further 250 by, for example, walking briskly for around 3 km (2 miles).

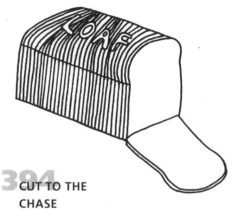

392 EAT SMALL TO EAT LESS

A lot of food satisfaction comes from how food looks on the plate, so to trick yourself into feeling satisfied with smaller portions, simply use smaller plates. It might sound silly, but studies have shown that people feel fuller if they think they've eaten a plateful, no matter what size!

393 EQUAL REWARDS

If you find overeating a problem, find a non-food alternative which you also find rewarding. This could include exercise, prayer, yoga, listening to music, browsing the internet, phoning a friend, reading a magazine, or many other alternatives.

394 CUT TO THE CHASE

If you're serving bread with a meal or in a sandwich, make sure you cut thin slices rather than doorsteps (thick slices). Most people will eat the same number of slices no matter how thick, so reduce calories by making slices thinner.

395 FULL STOP

Stop eating when you're full. It sounds simple, but many of us are conditioned to finish what's on our plates regardless of whether we've had enough. After every mouthful, pause and think about whether you really want the next one.

396 KEEP YOUR BALANCE

As a general guide for someone who does moderate exercise and isn't greatly over- or underweight, one pound of body fat equals 4000 calories. This means that in order to shed a pound a week, you would need to reduce your total number of calories by just over 500 calories a day.

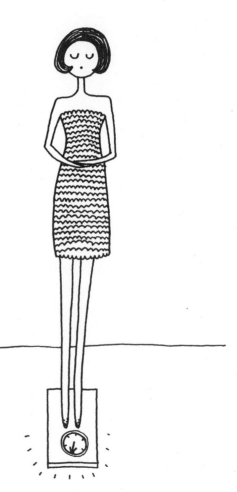

397 QUALITY NOT QUANTITY

The sight of a buffet table is enough to send most dieters running for cover, but don't despair – a good trick for keeping buffets healthy is to eat larger portions of fewer things, instead of lots of little nibbles. Pile up on protein, fruit and vegetables, and foods high in fibre.

398 LEAVE A NOTE

Many people snack on high-calorie foods without realising they're doing it. Train yourself out of it by leaving a note on the outside of your fridge to remind you that if you're going to have a snack you should a) want it and b) enjoy it.

399 SAVE YOURSELF FOR THE BEST

One useful guideline in cutting calories is that if it seems too good to be true, it probably is! Often, people who choose 'low fat' versions of their normal desserts or treats are disappointed when they just don't taste the same. Why not 'save up' your calories and have the occasional indulgent treat instead.

400 DIP YOUR NUTS

For a healthy after-dinner snack that won't pile on the pounds, choose nuts or dried fruits dipped in dark chocolate – at least 70% cocoa solids is best.

401 DITCH THE PASTRY

Quiche is often seen as a healthy choice, but the problem is the pastry. A standard 23-cm (9-inch) pastry case contains 41 g of fat, 63 g of carbohydrates and 818 mg of sodium. Choose a pastry-free omelette instead.

402 DIET WITH DAIRY

Calcium actually helps your body expel fat, helping you lose weight and maintain healthy cholesterol, but only if the calcium comes from dairy products. And lower-fat versions have the most absorbable minerals, so choose them where possible.

403 TRUST AN ANGEL

Instead of your usual afternoon cake or biscuits, try angel layer cake (or angel cake), which is much lower in fat. To make an even healthier snack, serve it with fruit purée.

404 A NEW COAT

If you're on a low-carb diet but want to make fish or chicken in breadcrumbs, try using crushed pork rinds instead, mixed with a few herbs or spices. That way, you'll get the crispy outer shell and stay carb-free.

405 SEE THROUGH SOUP

Instead of soups containing cream, choose those with tomato or clear broth as their base. So, instead of leek and potato or cream of mushroom, try tomato and herb or carrot and coriander.

406 MIX YOUR OWN YOGURTS

Replace fruit yogurts, which can contain quite high levels of sugar and fat, with your own fruit purée. Add it to low-fat natural yogurt and top with a sprinkling of seeds for an extra health boost.

407 GO FOR COTTAGE

Try puréeing low-fat cottage cheese into a smooth paste and using it instead of full-fat cream cheese in recipes and as a spread. Alternatively, combine half and half.

408 CHEESE MELT

If you're a toasted cheese sandwich fan but don't want the extra calories, make yourself a low-fat version by grilling the toast and adding a small amount of cheese which has been melted in the microwave. That way you cut down on non-essential fat.

409 CUT A QUARTER

When butter or oil is needed in recipes, try reducing the amount by a quarter. For instance, if your recipe calls for 50 g (2 oz) butter, try cutting it down to 25 g (1.5 oz). If you can't taste the difference, reduce it by another quarter next time. You will be surprised just how little fat is really necessary.

410 ROLL UP A TREAT

If you simply can't live without biscuits or cakes with your afternoon tea, choose healthier options. Fig rolls contain less saturated fat and more fruit content than chocolate biscuits or those with cream fillings. Mixed berry or fruit and spice oat biscuits have a low GI, too.

411 REAP THE REWARDS

Set yourself realistic goals and reward yourself (not with chocolate!) for achieving them. Try something like 'for one week I will eat one additional fruit or vegetable portion a day and avoid second helpings'.

412 MIST YOUR PAN

Instead of sloshing butter or margarine into the pan to prevent sticking while you're frying, invest in a plant mister and fill it with olive oil, which is a healthy cooking oil. Then, you can be sure you're only using as much as you really need.

413 SMOOTH OPERATOR

Thick smoothies can actually fill you up for longer than a solid meal because their volume causes the stomach to expand more. This makes them a great choice for breakfast or lunch, when you may have to wait some time before your next meal.

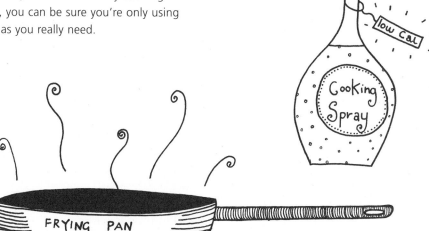

414 GRATE, FINE

It's the fat in cheese that helps it melt uniformly – low-fat varieties often melt in patches or take much longer. To make sure your low-fat cheese melts properly, grate it first using the fine side of your grater.

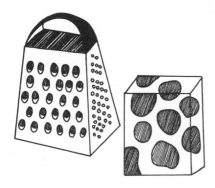

415 NO YOLKS PLEASE

An easy way to lower the calorie content of your egg sandwiches is to hard boil eggs and use only the egg whites for the filling. That way, you cut out on the calorific yolks but keep the eggy taste.

416 PICK LOW FAT

Instead of ice cream on desserts, choose low fat soya versions or simply use frozen yogurt for a yummy pudding without all the saturated fat or calories

417 DON'T BE A PRUNE PRUDE

If you're aiming for a calorie-controlled diet, try substituting prune paste for chocolate in recipes. The prunes taste sweet and have the added bonus of giving you a dose of healthy vitamins instead of the fat contained in chocolate.

counting calories

418 GO NAKED

If you're used to eating roast chicken with the skin on, removing the skin will reduce the calorie count from 220 to 155 for an average portion, as most of the fat is in the skin. Trim the calories further by removing any excess fat before cooking.

419 SWAP SHOP

Swap a bowl of normal ice cream (at 310 calories and 20 g fat) for low-fat frozen yogurt (at 200 calories and 2.5 g fat) – that's a saving of 110 calories and an astounding 17.5 g fat per serving! It tastes wonderful, too.

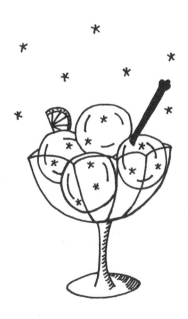

420 DRINK LIGHT

Choose light beer, which has an average of 95 calories per bottle, rather than the usual kind, which has around 150 calories. It might sound like a small saving, but if you're having it two or three times a week it could soon add up into a meaningful cut in the calorie count.

421 DILUTE YOUR DRINK

Alcohol adds many hidden calories – why not spread out your daily dose of wine into one or two spritzers and opt for low-calorie mixers where possible? You can save around 50 calories in a gin and tonic merely by switching to light tonic.

422 STAY LOW WITH H$_2$O

Liquid calories are digested much more quickly than solid, and provide a lot of extra calories without filling you up, which means it's likely you'll eat just as much food as you would without them. Two cups of fizzy drink each day is 220 calories, which is 10 kg (23 lb) in weight over a year. Water is the best option.

423 SKIM ON THE MILK

Each time you swap 1 cup of skimmed milk for one of whole milk, you'll save 70 calories. Based on one serving a day, at the end of the year you will save more than 25,000 calories and potentially lose 3 kg (7 lb).

424 SAY CHEESE

If you swap 30 g (1 oz) reduced-fat cheese (90 calories) for 30 g (1 oz) regular cheese (115 calories), you'll save 25 calories. And if you swap it for fat-free cheese you'll save 75 calories per ounce – perfect for sauces or pizza where the taste of the cheese isn't paramount.

425 PICK OF THE PIZZAS

If you want to add a serving of ice cream to your pizza meal, save the calories by choosing a vegetarian pizza over one with meat, which will reduce the calorie content from around 1,000 to 700, leaving you an extra 300 to finish your meal off in style!

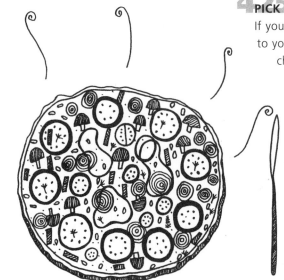

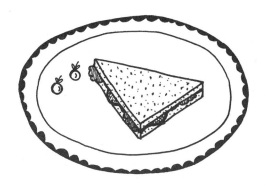

428 A HOT DATE

Instead of reaching for the chocolates after a meal, pop a date into your mouth. They contain much less sugar than chocolates and a range of health-giving vitamins and minerals, but still have a rich, sweet taste.

eating habits

429 SEE A PROFESSIONAL

If you're having trouble cutting sugary and fatty foods out of your diet, or you're trying to stick to a plan but the weight just isn't coming off, consider consulting a dietician. Most offer a one-off consultation that might help kick-start you into making some basic practical changes.

426 HALVE YOUR SANDWICH

Try opting for a half a sandwich at lunchtime, rather than your usual whole one – it's an easy way to halve your calories and you might find you feel just as full but less sluggish as a result.

427 THINK DRINKS

If you're trying to cut down on your calories, don't forget to count what you drink as well as what you eat. There are at least as many calories in the average can of fizzy drink as in a slice of cake.

430 STICK TO YOUR SIZE

One of the most dangerous temptations in dieting is the tendency to add a little bit more food. If you're on a calorie-restricted diet plan, make sure you stick strictly to portion sizes or weigh food carefully to avoid this common pitfall.

431 EAT TOGETHER

Try to get your whole family to sit down together for a meal at the table. It's thought that children from families who regularly eat together have healthier attitudes to food and are less likely to be obese than those who don't. Studies have shown that people who eat while watching TV eat more and enjoy their food less than those who sit at a table to eat.

432 BE PREPARED TO WORK

One of the most common reasons people reach for biscuits and other unhealthy snacks is that they're simply less work. Get ahead of yourself and spend 15 minutes or so peeling and chopping vegetables like carrots, fennel, cucumber, peppers and celery, or fruit such as apples and pears. Bag it all up and keep it in the fridge so you can reach for it whenever you want.

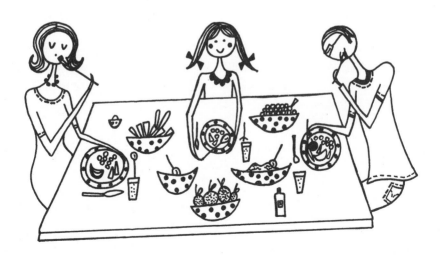

433 STICK TO THE SAME TIMES

If you often resort to snacking between meals, take a proactive step towards eliminating your bad habits by eating meals at regular times for a week. This will help keep calories more balanced and reduce hunger pangs and cravings.

434 EAT MORE OFTEN

If you find it hard not to snack between meals, eat more often – three meals a day doesn't suit everyone so try changing your routine to five or six smaller meals a day. For some people it's a way of eating that can help to keep blood sugar levels stable and keep you mentally alert and physically energetic all day long.

435 STOP BEFORE STUFFED

Try to eat until you are sufficiently satiated, rather than completely stuffed! In other words, try stopping when you feel 75–80% full and only eat more if you feel you really need to. To do this, you will have to learn to get 'in touch' with your feelings of hunger and fullness.

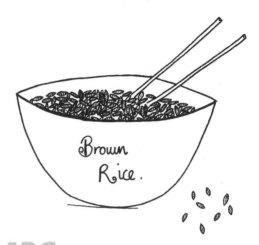

Brown Rice.

436 THE CHINESE WAY

Trick yourself into eating smaller portions of rice and noodle dishes by using chopsticks instead of a fork. The longer you take to eat, the more chance you give yourself to fill up before you've finished your plateful.

437 IN THE KITCHEN AT PARTIES

Many people find it difficult to control their eating at parties. As you arrive, take a look at the food and choose what you will eat. Fill up a plate rather than grazing at will, when you are much more likely to overeat.

438 KNOW YOUR WEAKNESS

If you know you have certain times of the day when you reach for snacks, try to pre-empt the problem by preparing a light meal or healthy snack ahead of time so you can reach for it when the craving strikes. Keep a bowl of fruit near your desk or on your kitchen table so you can pick from the bowl at any time during the day.

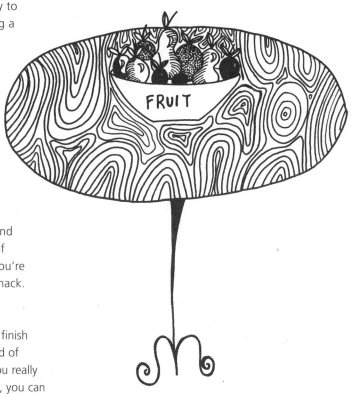

439 MORE THAN FOOD

To a lot of people, food isn't just food. Make a list of how you feel when you feel tempted to snack and what alternatives there might be. If you're bored, try changing what you're doing rather than reaching for a snack.

440 LEAVE SOMETHING BEHIND

For a week, make it a rule never to finish everything on your plate. At the end of the week, think back to whether you really noticed the difference. If you didn't, you can happily make your portions a little bit smaller.

441 COOK FROM SCRATCH

If you rely on fast foods or microwave meals, which are often high in saturated fat and added salt or sugar, try to make an effort to cook from scratch at least two or three nights a week instead. Switch one day at a time so you end up with only one or two processed-food days.

442 BECOME A COLLECTOR

Cooking for yourself, using fresh ingredients from scratch, doesn't have to be a long-winded affair. Collect a folder of ten-minute recipes and stock your cupboard accordingly so you're always prepared for those 'need-food-now' moments.

443 DO IT THE SLOW WAY

Calorie-controlled diets often work for a short time, but many people put on weight again after they stop, and they return to their old eating habits. Instead of dieting, cut calories every day in small ways, such as having fewer snacks and smaller portions. You'll lose weight more slowly but it's more likely to stay off.

444 WALK IT OFF

Make a point of going for a gentle walk after a meal, especially if you're eating out in the evening. Walking home instead of getting a taxi will help your meal 'settle' and can aid the digestive process.

445 SAVOUR THE FLAVOUR

Take a more Buddhist attitude to food by savouring every mouthful. Make yourself mindful of what you eat, what the flavours really taste like and how the food feels in your mouth. Pause after each mouthful and think about whether you really want more. Slowing down will make you feel fuller.

446 GET REGULAR

Eat regular meals – skipping meals can lead to hunger, often resulting in overeating. When you're very hungry your blood sugar levels plummet and it's tempting to forget about good nutrition. Snacking between meals can help curb hunger, but make sure the snack is healthy rather than high in fat or sugar – and don't eat so much that your snack becomes an entire meal.

447 START WITH JUICE

If you're used to knocking back a glass of wine as you cook, pour yourself a tomato juice instead, or even a glass of water, and drink that before you start on the alcohol. That way, you'll drink less and regulate your calorie intake.

448 FRUIT TEST

Some people find that eating fruit after a meal can cause bloating and gas problems – if you think fruit affects you in this way, try eating it an hour or two before or after a meal and see if it feels any different.

449 DRINK AWAY HUNGER

Are you really hungry – or dehydrated? Lack of water can make you think you're hungry for food, leading to overeating and weight gain. Cravings for salty foods are also a telltale sign of dehydration. Drink two litres of water daily at regular intervals.

450 THE ORIENTAL WAY

A great food to choose for working lunches is sushi, especially if you add a healthy salad or vegetable serving which will add some fibre to the meal. The fish will give you a boost of omega-3 oils to help brainpower, but make sure it's really fresh.

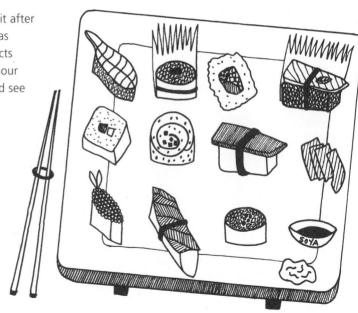

451 KEEP THE TREATS

Diets that cut out all 'treat' foods have been shown to be ineffective at keeping weight off in the long term. Instead, choose a healthy-eating style where you minimize (but don't cut out completely) unhealthy foods, replacing them with better choices. If nothing's forbidden, you won't be so tempted by it.

452 TIDY UP YOUR LEFTOVERS

Leaving food lying around is just too tempting – you might reach for a second helping – so put everything away as soon as you've served it.

453 STRESS FACTORS

Stress is often a trigger for eating – when we're stressed, not only are we likely to eat more, but we're more likely to go for the fast option as our bodies speed up. Our bodies can also crave certain types of food, such as those high in fats and sugars. Think about how this relates to your eating habits, and make changes in your life to reduce stress if necessary.

454 STOCK UP AT THE OFFICE

If you have a microwave in your office, stack your desk with some diet staples like individual packs of oatmeal and dried fruit – that way, you'll always be able to make yourself an energy-boosting, low-fat snack.

455 TAKE THE LONG VIEW

There will be times when you'll slip up and overeat or pick less healthy foods because they sound good, you're stressed or you just feel like it. Healthy eating is a lifelong goal and one slip up won't make any difference in the long run. If you overdo it one day, eat less the following day to redress the balance.

456 TOTAL YOUR DAY

Try and balance up your eating every day so that when you go to bed, you do it with a clean slate. For instance, if you have an unhealthy lunch or snack in the afternoon, make your evening meal a super-healthy salad with fish and fresh fruit. If the evening's been unhealthy, resolve to start afresh the next morning.

457 AGE BEFORE APPETITE

As you age, your metabolic rate changes as well as your lifestyle, so even active older people need fewer calories than when they were young. Alter your diet as you grow older by cutting down on fatty foods and making carbohydrate portions smaller.

458 TUNE IN

Eat when you're hungry, not just out of habit. Getting more in tune with your body's requirements will help you maintain healthy eating habits – by listening to what your body really needs instead of simply reaching for the biscuit tin every time you're bored, upset or angry.

459 DAY BY DAY

Make changes gradually and don't expect to totally revamp your eating habits overnight. Start to remedy excesses or deficiencies with modest changes, which will add up to create positive lifelong eating habits. For instance, if you don't like the taste of skimmed milk, try semi-skimmed; replace white rice with brown basmati, and so on.

460 MOVE ON

Be realistic about your target weight. It's likely to be unhealthy to aim to maintain your teenage weight as you get older, as your natural body weight increases with age as well as being affected by factors such as pregnancy. If you eat a healthy, balanced diet, the chances are your weight is fine.

461 LOOK AT YOUR FRAME

Don't be fooled by the media into thinking you should be thinner than is healthy – set yourself a sensible target weight which isn't hard to maintain with a healthy diet and normal levels of activity. If you often feel genuinely hungry or exercise too much, your target weight is probably too low.

462 DON'T DO A DIET

The word diet has negative connotations and can reduce body image – it's a sad fact that most people who admit to dieting don't manage to keep the weight off. Instead of concentrating on losing weight, make good health your aim.

463 KEEP A DIARY

If you've been trying to diet and not succeeding, try keeping a food diary for a week or two – write down everything you eat and drink. Seeing it in black and white can help you to identify vulnerable times of day, unhealthy eating patterns and areas you might not be aware of.

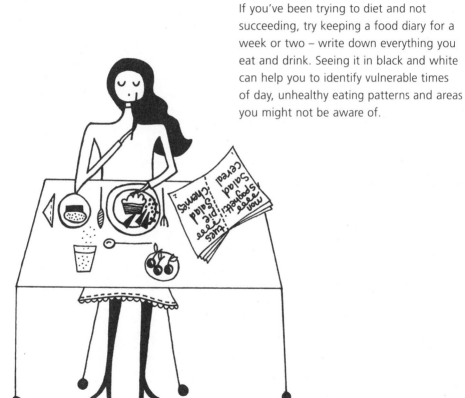

464 EXERCISE YOURSELF HAPPY

Studies have shown that one of the best ways to prevent overeating is to take regular exercise. This is because exercise releases feel-good endorphins in the body, and people who feel happier and more fulfilled are less likely to overeat.

465 ACTIVATE YOURSELF

Metabolism varies among individuals but only by up to 100 calories daily, so claiming a slow metabolism isn't an excuse for weight gain. Instead, look to the details of how you eat and how active you are, counting up hidden calories and making practical changes.

466 GET SOME THERAPY

If you feel your eating is out of control, or you struggle to implement changes for more than a few weeks at a time, perhaps it's time to consider some kind of behaviour therapy, which aims for gradual but permanent changes in behaviour alongside a sensible eating plan? Ask your doctor for advice on what kind of therapy or counselling to try.

467 SUMMER STRETCH

Throughout the summer, eat in line with the longer daylight hours so that your food intake is spread more evenly throughout the day. This usually means smaller, more frequent meals, which will make sense if it's hotter, too.

468 KNOW YOUR PITFALLS

To improve your eating habits, you first have to know what's wrong with them. Do you add a lot of butter, creamy sauces or salad dressings to your meals? Rather than eliminating them completely, just cut back your portions instead.

469 YOUR OWN JUDGE

Don't let other people determine how much you eat. Ask to serve yourself if you're out, and don't listen to friends or colleagues who say you should eat more or less. Be your own judge of what's a healthy portion for you.

470 EAT WHEN ALERT

Don't eat first thing in the morning, before you are fully awake, or last thing at night because your mind is not alert at these times and you might overeat without meaning to.

food philosophy

471 PORTION PICKER

Studies have shown that people given larger portions eat more no matter how hungry they feel. Instead of serving dinner on to plates, which means one person is deciding the portion sizes, serve foods in bowls on the table and allow everyone to take as little or as much as they want.

472 DIET DETOURS

A cake here and missed workout there – it happens! Don't starve or punish yourself in any other way to try to compensate if you slip up. It's much healthier for your brain and body – and you're much more likely to continue the diet successfully – if you let it go rather than prolonging feelings of guilt.

473 COLOUR COORDINATE

The way food looks can be as important as how it tastes in the satisfaction ratings. Help yourself enjoy your food more by taking a few minutes to make sure it's well presented on the plate.

474 LONG-TERM COMMITMENT

Dedicate some time to making long-term changes in the way you and your family eat. Every time you go to the supermarket, swap one of your usual unhealthy food choices – like a packet of biscuits – for a healthy choice such as dried fruit or oatcakes. That way, you're more likely to keep up the healthy changes.

475 GIVE TASTE A CHANCE

Because processed foods often have stronger tastes than freshly cooked meals, your tastebuds can become used to them. If you cut them out, flavours that used to seem appetizing may well lose their appeal as your palate regains its sensitivity and you start to appreciate tastes more.

476 FOCUS ON FLAVOUR

Don't forget to taste your food. It may sound ridiculous, but many people – especially those prone to overeating or comfort snacking – get satisfaction from eating rather than actual food. Engage the senses in the pleasure of eating.

477 STAY STABLE

Excess body fat increases your chances of high blood pressure, heart disease, stroke, diabetes, some types of cancer and other illnesses. But being too thin can increase your risk of osteoporosis, menstrual irregularities and other health problems. The worst from a health point of view, however, is to fluctuate between the two. Aim to find a stable weight and stay there.

478 GET SOME SATISFACTION

Foods that fill you up best and reduce hunger pangs are those that are high in protein. Fish and skinless chicken are good examples, and to feel most satisfied you should aim to include a serving of these foods in each meal.

479 SLOWLY DOES IT

If you feel you've lost touch with the enjoyment of eating, consider joining the Slow Food organisation, a global movement that's dedicated to encouraging people to reconnect with the pleasure of eating healthy, wholesome foods.

480 EAT BLINDFOLDED

If you worry about overeating and can't seem to tell when you're full, try eating blindfolded! Studies have shown that people eat 25% less food when blindfolded and feel fuller more quickly. Just make sure your plate is to hand and not the cat's dinner!

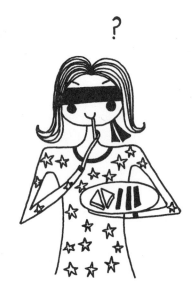

481 PLATE MATES

Did you know you're more likely to feel satisfied after a meal if you've finished a full plate of food? A simple and effective way to reduce your portion size, and still feel full, is to trick yourself into eating smaller portions by buying smaller plates.

482 ADJUST YOUR ATTITUDE

Understanding your food psychology can help you gain control over your eating. Every few months, make time to sit down and think about your attitudes to food. Include things like how you ate as a child and how you feel when you overeat, and use these insights to help you change your eating habits. Many unhealthy eating behaviours are simply bad habits.

483 LIMIT THE CHOICE

We tend to eat more when our eyes tell our brains that there's lots of variety to choose from. Cut back on the choice available and serve food on one large platter instead of several small ones; studies have shown that you will eat less overall.

484 DON'T PULL THE TRIGGER

Appetite can be affected by certain foods, which trigger good memories and cause the release of chemical messages to the brain – which in turn trigger the stomach to feel hungry. If you understand your trigger foods, it might be possible to intercept this process before hunger strikes, and to avoid them.

485 GIVE YOURSELF A MINI-BREAK

Psychologically, you're more likely to stop snacking if you have to keep opening new packets. If overeating is a problem for you, consider buying mini-portions of your favourite snacks – opening each one as you eat it and collecting a pile of wrappers will help you limit intake.

486 CHOOSE A BOWL

If you're eating a stackable food like pasta, rice or noodles, eat from a bowl rather than a plate to help you feel fuller quicker. Eating a pile of food rather than one spread out on a plate tricks the body into thinking it's eaten more.

487 MAKE IT A TALL ONE

Our brain tends to recognize height quicker than width. If you drink from a tall thin glass as opposed to a short fat one, your brain will think you're having more even if you drink the same amount.

488 BE REALISTIC

Sometimes you'll still have a take-away, a burger, a ready-meal, or simply not be able to resist the allure of deep fried crisps, chips or creamy desserts. Relax and enjoy it – healthy eating is all about balance and as long as you're eating well most of the time, it's fine to give in occasionally.

489 TAKE STEPS

If you've recognised that your eating has emotional cues, put in place some steps to allow you to take control – Stop, Breathe, Reflect (on why you're about to eat) and Choose (to eat the food, not eat it, eat half of it, eat an alternative, and so on). Get into the habit of doing this whenever you feel the impulse to reach for food outside mealtimes.

490 DARE TO BE DIFFERENT

Eat differently, not less. Instead of your next serving of pasta, bread or rice, try a large portion of mixed salad. A full plate of salad is physically and psychologically filling, but contains few calories and plenty of vitamins and minerals.

491 ASK YOURSELF A QUESTION

Before you reach for that sugary snack, ask yourself, 'If I eat this food now, is it worth it?' These questions bring mindfulness to eating rather than just doing it on impulse or obeying urges. It doesn't guarantee the eating won't happen – it just gives you a chance to make a better decision.

492 LOOK AT THE LABEL

Use food labels to create balance and diversity in your diet (see Understanding Labels, page 8). By looking at the labels and learning to understand them, you can include less healthy foods in your diet as long as they are balanced with foods that are healthier. This will help you to keep to your recommended daily amounts.

healthy snacking

493 AU NATURAL

If you're a fan of peanut butter, but not of the high levels of unhealthy trans fats – which can't be properly digested by the body – it contains, switch to a natural product. While no lower in calories, these are free of hydrogenated oils. Great spread on crackers or oatcakes and eaten with an apple as a mid-morning snack.

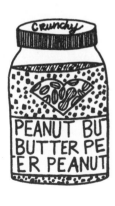
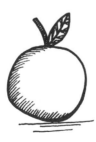

494 CARE FOR CAROB

If you want an alternative to caffeine-rich chocolate that is cocoa and dairy free, try chocolate substitutes made with the tree bark of the carob tree. These taste naturally sweet and so will contain quite a lot less sugar than many chocolate bars.

495 CUT THE CHEESE CONTENT

Instead of smothering your pizza or salad with lots of high-fat low-flavour cheese, switch to a highly flavoured cheese like Parmesan, extra mature Cheddar or a blue cheese such as Stilton or Gorgonzola, and use a smaller amount. A tablespoon of Parmesan contains only 2 g of fat (one of which is saturates).

496 SERVICE-STATION TRAP

Car journeys can be long and you might find yourself eating to keep awake. And, of course, service stations are waiting for you with a tempting array of super-sized snacks. To avoid the temptation, set off on your journey with a good choice of healthy snacks to see you through.

497 STAY WELL STOCKED

Lots of people get hungry for sugary snacks in the evening, and if you're at home watching TV it can be difficult to resist that bar of chocolate. Keep healthy snacks to hand – low-fat yogurt, dried or fresh dates, figs or mango, oatcakes – and only have the chocolate if you still want it after you've had two healthy snacks.

498 KEEP IT FRESH

All fruit is healthy but dried fruit is significantly higher in calories than fresh fruit. This is because the moisture is taken out, leaving more sugar per serving. If you're trying to lose weight, it's best to stick to fresh fruit, which you can eat more of for the same number of calories.

499 ON THE MOVE

Next time you reach for a snack when you're out shopping or in the car, stop and think whether you're really hungry. Are you bored, tired? Does it just happen to be there? Carry a healthy snack such as nuts or oatcakes in your bag for times like this.

500 LOOK BELOW THE SURFACE

Don't be fooled into thinking yogurt-coated nuts and raisins are healthy foods. They are filled with calories, sugar and fat without any of the active cultures of fresh yogurt, In fact, the yogurt taste is often just flavouring. Just 20 yogurt-covered nuts provide around 460 calories, 32 g fat and 8 tsp sugar. Instead, choose nuts in the shell – they will take longer to eat, giving your brain more time to recognize you are full.

501 AIR-POPPED CORN

Popcorn is a great filler and fibre provider and has only 100 calories and 3.5 g fibre per regular serving – much less than nuts and dried fruit. But choose air-popped corn rather than fried, and don't add lashings of salty or sweet toppings.

502 CUT THE COFFEE

There might be a coffee bar on every street corner, but that doesn't mean you need to stop for a top-up at every one! Coffee drinks can be really high in fat and calories because of the milk and syrup – mocha coffee has 11 g fat, cappuccino 6 g and regular white coffee 1 g fat, so choose carefully – and don't dip in a sweet snack.

503 IT HAD BETTER BE CELERY

Celery is a super snack food – not only is it crunchy and refreshing, it genuinely does take your body the same amount of calories to eat and digest it as it gives you. Avoid smothering it with creamy dips and go for healthy versions instead, such as hummus made with olive oil or low-fat yogurt mixed with garlic and fresh herbs.

504 SERVE YOURSELF A SALAD

So that you've always got a healthy option when you open the fridge door, make up a large bowl of salad a couple of times a week and get into the habit of serving it with every meal, adding extra vegetables to your diet.

505 CHOOSE DECAF

Many people swear by the caffeine in tea, coffee, chocolate and many soft drinks to give them a boost whenever they're flagging, but caffeine addiction can lead to fatigue and lack of concentration. Give yourself a break for a few days or switch to decaffeinated drinks – even if just a cup or two a day.

506 FISHY PÂTÉ

To help you get your extra portions of fish, make your own fish pâté using canned fish with your favourite sauce – think horseradish with salmon and mackerel, or tomato with tuna – to use as a sandwich spread during the week.

507 KEEP IT INDIVIDUAL

Never take a whole box or packet of snacks or food to eat in front of the computer, television or while reading, because you might absentmindedly eat more than you intend. Serve yourself an individual portion in a bowl instead, and get yourself a refill only if you really want more.

508 DANGER ZONES

Most people have 'danger times' for snacking during the day (for a lot of women it's around 4 pm). Make an effort not to be around fatty snacks at this time, or take along a healthier alternative such as nuts and seeds.

509 GRAB A GRAPE

Keep a bunch of grapes in your fridge and grab a handful when you fancy something sweet. They release sugar quickly, so are great for satisfying cravings – wait ten minutes and only reach for the chocolate if the grapes really don't hit the spot.

510 CAN YOU BURN IF OFF?

For each pound of body weight you want to burn off, you need to use up roughly 3500 calories, so unless you're about to become a marathon runner, think carefully about which snacks you choose.

511 UP WATER LEVELS

Drinking water is essential for keeping your system healthy – not only does it keep your cells hydrated and help your organs function optimally, it also keeps food flowing through the digestive system, which means you'll derive more benefits from your healthy foods.

512 SUGAR-FREE YOUR IMMUNITY

Cutting down on snack foods containing refined sugar can limit your susceptibility to fatigue, colds and winter bugs. High levels of sugar affect immunity by reducing the efficiency of white blood cells.

513 LOW-CAL YOUR HOT DRINKS

Try using skimmed, or fat-free, milk instead of your usual whole or semi-skimmed version in hot drinks where calories can add up without you realizing. This could save you 30 calories per cup of tea or filter coffee, even more if you drink cappuccino or latte. And ditch the syrups and flavourings.

514 GO BANANAS

For an energy boost to help you through a late-afternoon dip in energy, choose a banana. They're packed with potassium for extra energy.

515 PACK UP THE CAR

If car journeys are a time you find it difficult not to snack, pre-empt your cravings by packing fruit and vegetables in snack-sized portions, or healthy rice cakes or dried fruits. Pack enough for the family, so you won't be tempted by their snacks.

eating out

516 STICK TO THE RULES

Keep to the ground rules wherever you are. Whether you're eating at home or eating out, make efforts to apply the principles of healthy nutrition by eating a variety of healthy foods, limiting fat, sugar and salt, and keeping portion sizes in check.

517 SIZE MATTERS

Be aware of portion size when eating out – if the restaurant offers meals in several sizes, choose the smallest. Or get creative and order two starters or a child-sized meal. You can also share meals or ask the restaurant to put half the meal in a take-away container before it's served.

518 DON'T BE SHY

Never feel like you're stepping out of line if you request healthier options or substitutions in a restaurant, pub or bar. You're not being difficult, so don't be swayed – you're simply doing what it takes to stay committed to your healthy-eating plan.

519 NO SKIPPING

Don't be sucked into the false economy of starving yourself at lunchtime if you know you're going out in the evening. Being hungry will just make you eat more, and you'll be more likely to reach for unhealthy snacks. Choose healthy, filling foods such as vegetable soup with lentils or beans, or a baked sweet potato.

520 STICK TO THE ROUTINE

Try to keep to regular mealtimes, even if you're eating out, to help you ward off food cravings and keep your blood-sugar levels regular. If you're booking a table for lunch or dinner, book it for your usual eating time rather than forcing your body to wait until later.

521 TWO FORKS ARE BETTER THAN NONE

Next time you're tempted by a calorie-packed pudding at a restaurant, why not share instead of having a whole one to yourself. It will give you the benefit of all the taste with half the calories. You just need to find a willing partner!

522 SALAD DAYS

Don't be fooled into thinking all salads are healthy. For instance, thanks to excessive dressing, croutons and added cheese, a standard chicken Caesar salad can total 1130 calories and add more than 90 g of fat to your diet! Make it healthier by cutting out the croutons and dressing with a small amount of vinaigrette.

523 ASK FOR ADVICE

Don't be afraid to ask for advice in a restaurant. If you're worried about which dishes contain more fat or calories, ask the waiting staff. Or tell them you're cutting calories and ask the chef to recommend the best option.

524 NO NEED TO VEGETATE

Don't use your dietary limitations as an excuse not to venture out to eat – even restaurants that don't offer vegan options can usually whip up a meatless pasta or vegetable plate if you ask. Ask the waiting staff or phone ahead and speak to the manager or chef directly.

525 DON'T BLOW IT

Having a light snack, such as wholemeal toast, a banana or a low-calorie yogurt before you go out to dinner will take the edge off hunger and stop you gorging on the bread basket the minute you sit down. Make it a low-sugar wholegrain snack, or have a glass of skimmed milk.

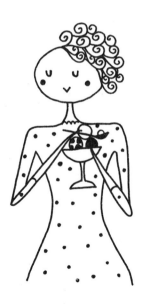

526 SWAP FAT FOR FIBRE

Try to swap high fat foods for low fat, high fibre wherever you can. For instance, instead of roast or fried potatoes with your meal, ask for extra vegetables or salad instead. Most restaurants are used to catering for a range of dietary requirements so these types of request aren't rare.

527 HALF AND HALF

Make your food choice healthier by swapping half the meat for low-fat vegetarian options such as thick slices of marinated tomato, courgette or aubergine. Serve with buns instead of meat or with burgers as a cheese alternative.

528 A FORK FULL

If you want the taste of salad dressing with out the extra calories, try the fork method – order dressing on the side and dip your fork into it before each mouthful. It might sound silly, but most restaurant salads are overdressed, and this is away of making sure you only get as much as you want and consume fewer calories.

528 BREAD WARNING

In restaurants, filling up on bread before your meal starts is a hidden danger, especially as you're likely to be eating more than normal anyway. Choose grain breads wherever you can, share with someone else and eat without butter to minimize health costs.

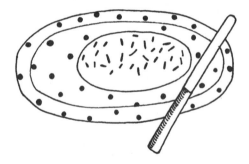

530 WORLD-WISE

Trying different world foods is a great way to make changes to your diet – experiment with different flavours and amalgamate those you like into your diet.

531 FRUIT DESSERTS

If you're eating out, try to choose desserts containing fruit whenever possible. Even higher-fat options such as apple crumble and fruit tarts usually contain fewer calories than non-fruit cakes and creamy puddings.

532 BE CORDIAL

Instead of fizzy drinks, which can contain lots of additives and sugar, and therefore be high in calories, try mixing sparkling mineral water with a fruit juice or cordial for a much healthier flavoursome drink.

533 THINK THIN

If you're out at a pizza restaurant, steer clear of thick and stuffed crusts, which contain hidden calories. Instead, go for the traditional Italian thin-crust version, which contains less fat and carbohydrate.

534 END WITH A SALAD

If you want pudding but you don't want to ruin your healthy eating plan, choose a healthy fruit salad or a sorbet, which are lower in calories than other puddings.

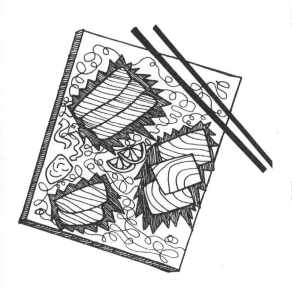

536 PLAN AHEAD

If you have to entertain or eat out a lot for your work, organize your week in advance and try to have only one function a day where you'll allow yourself to be tempted by unhealthy food, and don't have too much of it. Give yourself one or two occasions a week to relax and blow out and stick to healthy options for the rest.

537 OIL-LESS

When ordering grilled fish or vegetables in restaurants, ask that the food either be grilled without butter or oil, or prepared light, with less oil or butter than would usually be used.

535 CHOOSE SASHIMI

A great food to choose for working lunches is sashimi, especially if you add a healthy salad or vegetable serving to add some fibre to the meal. The fish will give you a boost of omega-3 oils to help brainpower when you get back to work, but make sure it's really fresh.

538 GET REAL

It's time to make some changes to your attitude towards eating out – with today's modern lifestyles, eating out is more a part of life than a special occasion for many, which means you can't always use it as an excuse to let go. Be realistic about how often you eat out and think about how to include it in your lifestyle changes.

539 PLUMP FOR TOMATO

When ordering pasta and rice dishes, look for tomato-based sauces rather than cream-based ones because they are much lower in fat and calories. And the tomato in the sauce counts as one of your five-a-day, so you can tuck in guilt-free!

540 SEE THE WHOLE

Think of eating out in the context of your whole healthy-eating plan. If it's a special occasion that simply won't be the same without your favourite foods, go for it. Moderation is the general rule but as long as it doesn't become a habit, a bit of excess now and again is fine. Remember not to starve yourself in advance as it leads to bingeing and overeating.

541 START WITH A SOUP

Soups are a great starter choice because most are lower in calories than the other menu options and will fill you up more, so you eat less. Choose a clear soup and bear in mind that cream-based soups are higher in fat and calories than most other soups.

542 BRING ON A SUBSTITUTE

If you're eating out late and you don't want to eat too many carbohydrates, ask if your starch serving can be replaced with extra steamed vegetables.

543 PEER PRESSURE

If you're out with friends and it looks like everyone's having a starter, don't feel pressured into it unless you want to. You could always ask if anyone wants to share one with you to limit your intake.

544 MASH UP A SIDE DISH

If you have a choice of side dishes, opt for baked or mashed potato rather than chips. Even if these choices are not listed, you can ask if there are other options or request vegetables instead.

545 HOLD BACK

Try not to eat out in 'eat as much as you like' restaurants, or those with buffet-only choices. You are more likely to overfill your plate and overeat in these places than when ordering from a menu.

546 LOSE THE FAT (BUT KEEP THE TOYS)

Children love the kid's meal offered in restaurants – more for the fun box and toys than for the food. Let them order the kid's meal, but ask for substitutions for the unhealthy fizzy drinks and chips (fries).

547 ON THE SIDE

Often, restaurants smother salad in dressing, giving you far more oil that you would choose at home. Order the dressing in a jug on the side and you can be sure you only use as much as you need.

548 NO MORE FRY-UPS

Look for items on the menu that are baked, grilled, dry-sautéed, broiled, poached or steamed as these cooking techniques use less fat in the food preparation and are generally lower in calories. Steer clear of deep-fried foods.

549 GO LIGHT ON CHEESE

When you're ordering a meal containing cheese in a restaurant, ask the chef to make it light on the cheese – you'll still get the cheesy taste without all the added calories.

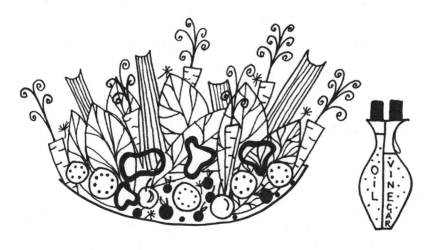

550 A HEALTHY CHOICE

Many restaurants indicate healthy choices on their menus, and most sit-down places will modify menu items on your request. Additionally, fast-food restaurants now offer a wider range of healthy choices and most will provide nutritional information if asked, or you can check it on their websites in advance.

551 LEAVE A THIRD

Portion sizes in restaurants are usually at least double what a person would normally eat, especially as you usually have more than one course, so it is important to keep that in mind when ordering and eating. If your portion is too large, a good rule of thumb is to leave a third of each serving.

552 BEFORE-DESSERT COFFEE

Try ordering your tea or coffee before dessert rather than at the end of your meal. After you've drunk it, the rest of your meal will have had 20 minutes or so to settle and make you feel full, and you're less likely to want to order dessert.

553 AN EYE ON THE ALCOHOL

One of the ways extra calories slip in to meals is with high-calorie alcohol – don't allow yourself to lose track of how much you're drinking. Empty your glass before you accept a top up and try to stick to one or two glasses per meal, alternating with a glass of water. Look out for low-calorie mixers and drink spritzers.

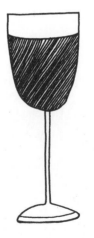
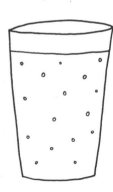

554 ENJOY YOUR EATING

Whatever you do, don't let healthy eating ruin your meal out – if you're in danger of letting calorie-reduction tips overwhelm you, stick to one or two tips, and if you do it often enough they will become habits.

555 MAKE A RULE OF TWO

Make a rule of eating only two courses – choose either a starter or a pudding, but don't have all three courses. Check the menu and see what really takes your fancy, then choose your tastiest meal.

556 LET YOURSELF FILL UP

It takes 20 minutes for our stomach to send the message to our brain that we're full, so make sure you take the time to chew and taste your food to avoid overeating.

557 LIMIT YOUR OUTINGS

Limit the amount of times you and your family eat out each week. Studies have shown that children and teenagers consume nearly twice as many calories and more fat when they eat out than at home.

558 A LA CARTE

It's usually a good idea to stick to the à la carte menu rather than fixed menus. The portion sizes are usually slightly smaller – and the chef will be more receptive to you asking for changes.

fast food & take-aways

559 SIZE UP THE PORTION

If you're ordering fast food, make sure your portion hasn't been supersized without you realizing. Many restaurants will assume you want more food for the same price. If unsure, ask for a regular or medium size.

560 HALF AT A TIME

Pre-made sandwiches in supermarkets are often designed for the hungriest people. Be aware of how much you eat by serving yourself one half at a time and only starting the second half if you are hungry.

561 AVOID UNREFINED

Subjecting foods to processing and refining, often at high temperatures, is a very effective way of robbing them of any nutritional value they might have originally possessed. Some processed foods have added vitamins and minerals but others have none at all. It's best to avoid them.

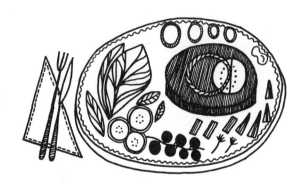

562 TAKE IT AWAY

Order food to take away rather than eating in fast-food restaurants as studies show that people tend to consume more food when they are not eating at their own table. Plus, you also have the option of providing a healthier side dish such as fruit or vegetables.

563 DELI-BELLY

If you're heading out for fast food, choose the deli-style shops and counters rather than pre-made options. Staff are more likely to take into account your requests to make your choice healthier, such as reducing butter or mayonnaise, and they're usually made with fresher ingredients.

564 BUN OFF

If you're eating out at a burger joint, reduce the amount of refined carbohydrates and calories in your meal by removing the top half of your burger bun and eating it with a knife and fork. Ask for a salad rather than fries, but keep the cheese and tomato.

565 CHOP THE CHINESE

Next time you reach for the phone to order that Chinese takeaway meal, be aware that the average take-away contains a whopping 1,000 calories, which means it's likely to be around half of your daily intake. And that's before pudding!

566 A SHAKY CHOICE

Milk shakes might sound like a healthy option, and they are if you make them at home with skimmed or semi-skimmed milk and fresh fruit. However, in restaurants they are usually made with full fat milk, sugary fruit syrup and flavourings – in which case they're not a good choice. Far better to have water or a smoothie if they're on offer.

567 A LIGHTER OPTION

Most fast-food establishments now offer healthier menu options such as soups, salads, sushi, chicken sandwiches and non-meat hamburgers. Choose these lighter options if you're in a rush and need to buy something to eat on the go.

568 VEGGIE BURGER SUBSTITUTE

Next time you're tempted by a burger – which is high in saturated fat as well as salt, and may not be made from good-quality meat – order a vegetarian version instead. With the same sauces it's often hard to taste the difference, and it's much better for you.

569 WHAT'S NOT THERE

It's not just what's in fast foods that's alarming. What they leave out – vitamins, minerals and fibre, to name a few – has just as bad an impact on your health and your digestive system, slowing it down and causing ill health and fatigue.

570 DON'T CUT THE MUSTARD

Choose mustard instead of mayonnaise on restaurant or fast food meals to cut calories by reducing fat. If your fast food option is pre-made with lots of mayonnaise, get the same effect by scraping off the excess.

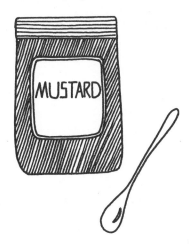

571 GRILL YOUR BIRD

Chicken is a great source of protein but it's not always the healthiest menu choice – make sure you choose grilled chicken pieces rather than those which are fried or breaded, and don't go for food like nuggets unless you are sure they're made with real chicken meat.

572 BEWARE OF BIG

In recent years, the portion size of salty snacks like crisps has increased by 93 calories, soft drinks by 49 calories and chips by 68 calories, so you're getting more than you used to even if you order the same thing. Check the labels when you're choosing unhealthy snacks.

573 CURRY'S FINE

Don't think you can't have a curry on your healthy eating plan – curries can be fattening but there are ways around it. Simply choose plain boiled rice over fried and opt for dry meats (like tandoori) instead of those with creamy sauces. Add a vegetable dish like dahl instead of oily bread.

574 FISHY FRIDAYS

One of the UK's favourite take-away meals is fish and chips – far from being banned from healthy-eating lists, it's much better news than many Chinese or Indian alternatives. To make it healthy, go small on chips, or remove them altogether, and replace with a salad at home.

575 LOOK FOR REPLACEMENTS

Don't settle for what comes with your sandwich or meal without considering a healthy option. Instead of chips, choose a healthy side salad or fruit bowl, and ask for salsa or tomato-based sauces instead of cheese and mayonnaise.

family food

576 INVOLVE THE KIDS

Do encourage your children to be involved in choosing and preparing food from an early age – that way, they're more likely to develop a healthy attitude to food that will last them a lifetime.

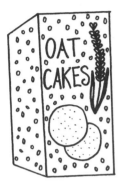

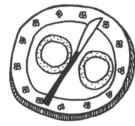

578 SUGAR HIT

Many parents worry that their children's behaviour will be adversely affected by foods containing lots of sugar at parties, but some studies have shown that hyperactivity is more likely to be caused by overstimulation. Either way, let them blow out once in a while.

579 VEG SUBSTITUTE

Rice salads made with brown rice or pasta salads of wholewheat pasta are great choices for healthy lunches for kids. If you struggle to get your kids to eat brown rice, don't despair – simply cut down on the white rice and add extra chopped vegetables for fibre instead.

577 LET THEM EAT OATCAKE

Oatcakes are great fibre-filled additions to healthy lunchboxes, as are rice cakes, especially the wholegrain ones, and corn cakes. These foods also make great travelling snacks as they are easily transported and children like them. Avoid those that are flavoured as they're usually coated with salty flavourings, and choose low-salt varieties where you can.

580 LEAD BY EXAMPLE

The best way to help your family adopt healthy eating habits is to have them yourself. It's hard for children to eat healthily if they see you snacking on high fat, sugar or salt foods. Try new fruits and vegetables and set a routine for your meals and snacks that they can follow.

581 CUT OUT THE WHITE

Buy seed- or oat-topped wholemeal rolls, wholemeal breads with poppyseeds or nuts (if allowed – some schools don't allow nuts because of allergies) or wholemeal pittas for your children's lunchbox instead of overprocessed white bread.

582 SUGAR TRAP

Yogurts and fromage frais are popular with most kids but many – especially the tubed varieties which are so easy to eat – are sugar-laden, with even a mini-pot containing more than 1 tsp of sugar and little or no real fruit. Limit the amount your children eat, or give them sugar-free or natural yogurt, with fresh fruit on the side.

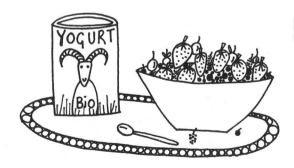

583 JOBS FOR TEENS

Give your teenagers some autonomy in the kitchen by taking a night off and allocating them one night a week to make the family meal. That way, they'll learn to cook for themselves before they leave home, and hopefully they'll enjoy planning and preparing a healthy meal.

584 A BALANCED LUNCHBOX

In a recent UK government survey, the contents of 74% of lunchboxes for kids were below the nutritional standards set for school meals. For a child aged 9–12 lunch should provide 585 kcal of energy, 23.7 g of fat (of which 7.5 g saturates), 81.3 g of carbohydrate and no more than 1.83 g of salt.

585 TEETHING PROBLEMS

Many baby biscuits and toddler's teething rusks contain sugar, which can damage baby's teeth before they've even emerged properly! Check labels carefully and choose biscuits sweetened with natural fruit juices – such as apple or grape – instead.

586 VITAL VITAMINS

Children need certain vitamins to keep their concentration levels high at school, and some – such as B-vitamins, vitamin C and particularly vitamin E, have been shown to help correct some behavioural problems. Supplements are useful, but vitamins from food are always best.

587 BREAK OUT THE BROWN

Sandwiches are a great lunchbox favourite but kids often prefer white bread, which isn't as good for them as wholemeal varieties. Try making their sandwiches with one slice of wholemeal and one of white, but remember to put the white slice on top so it's the one they see first.

588 CHOOSE CHEESE FOR SNACKS

Cheese is an excellent snack food for children, but beware of the snack-size individually wrapped versions, which can contain more salt than if they're cut from a bigger block. Check the label and if in doubt, pack a wrapped finger of ordinary cheese instead.

589 CAN'T BEAT A BANANA

Bananas are a great snack food and perfect for lunchboxes but they can often get bruised by vigorous movement! Invest in a Banana Guard for your child, a plastic housing which will keep the banana bruise-free until lunchtime!

590 GREEN UP YOUR SARNIES

Make yourself a rule for your children's sandwiches – never let a sandwich leave your home unless it's got some greenery in it. Spinach, lettuce, spring greens and watercress are all good sandwich fillers, and if you cut it up small, they'll probably get bored before they can pick it all out!

591 DRINK UP

Water is always the best drink for kids. Your children should always have access to water, and should have more water than any other drink during the day. If they're not keen on plain water, try sparkling mineral water for special occasions, or add a slice of lemon or lime or a dash of pure fruit juice for flavour.

592 STIR UP A SOUP

Soup is lovely in winter, and you can use just about any combination of vegetables to make it. Heat to just below boiling, pour it into a small, warmed flask and it'll be just the right temperature by the time you get to lunch. It's also a great choice for children's lunchboxes.

593 MILK THE HEALTH BENEFITS

Plain milk is a great choice for kids, because it contains essential vitamins and minerals and doesn't cause tooth decay. Children up to the age of two years should drink whole milk for the extra calories. After that they can move on to semi-skimmed, but don't give skimmed milk until children are at least five years old.

594 A GOOD CHEESE

'Lite' versions of cheese may be lower in fat than the original but, unbelievably, they sometimes contain sugar, so it's important you check labels carefully. Spreads do too. You're probably better off with half the amount of your normal cheese.

595 OFFER AN OLIVE

Olives are a great snack for children as they are healthy snacks – filling and without sugar or fat. They can be salty, though, if stored in brine, so wash before eating or offer water alongside them.

596 TAKE A DIP

Children love the process of dipping into sauces, so give them a sauce or dip they love, then slip some raw vegetables – sugar snap peas, carrot sticks, celery or peppers – into their hand and they'll (hopefully) eat them without fuss.

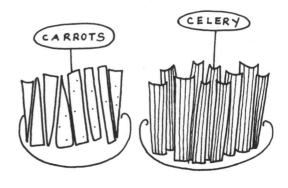

587 SMUGGLE SOME VEG

Sandwiches, rolls, pizzas and pitta breads are a great place to hide vegetables to help your kids get their five a day. Try grated carrots, finely chopped peppers, sliced cucumber and shredded greens.

588 EAT, DRINK AND BE HEALTHY

Try to limit your children's intake of drinks that may contain sugar – like fizzy drinks, fruit squashes and cordials – to mealtimes only as they often contain high amounts of sugar, which is healthier for teeth if taken with food and in one go rather than in little bits. Opt for low sugar or high juice varieties if you can.

589 A REAL SMOOTHIE

If you're struggling to get your children to eat their five portions of fruit and vegetables a day, remember smoothies! Homemade, they are a great way of tricking your kids into eating healthily, especially if made with live yogurt. If you buy them, make sure you choose those made with real fruit rather than concentrate.

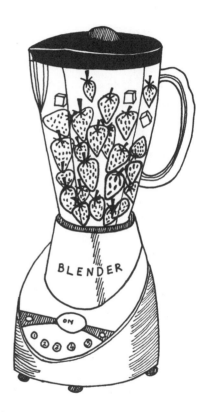

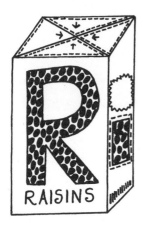

RAISINS

600 DRIED UP

For healthy family or kid's snacks, try dried fruits like raisins, apricots or prunes, which are sweet in taste because of the natural fructose sugars they contain but which also provide a healthy vitamin and mineral boost.

601 DRINK TIMES

Juices are' best drunk at mealtimes, and not sipped throughout the day, when they're more likely to damage teeth. Limit children to the one glass of pure fruit juice a day that counts towards their five portions of fruit and veg.

602 SEASONAL SHOPPING

Whenever you can, buy fresh fruits that are in season like apples, cherries, strawberries or peaches to use for snacks for your children. Cut them up into bite-sized pieces and put in small ziplock bags or plastic pots for easy snacking.

603 KEEP KIDS SALT FREE

It's important to ensure children don't have too much salt. While adults should have no more than 6 g of salt a day, children need even less as they have smaller bodies and less-developed organs. Check processed foods such as crisps, ready meals and sauces, even breakfast cereals, including those aimed at children. Opt for those with the least sodium.

604 SAFE SALT LEVELS

As a general rule, the maximum amounts of salt children should have at different ages are 2 g a day (0.8 g sodium) aged 1–3; 3 g a day (1.2 g sodium) aged 4–6; 5 g a day (2 g sodium) aged 7-10; and 6 g a day (2.5 g sodium) aged 11 and over.

605 PACK A HEALTHY PUNCH

In the UK, around half of all children take packed lunches to school, totalling 5.5 billion lunches a year, but it's estimated that less than half contain fruit and nine out of ten contain foods that are high in sugar, salt and saturated fat. Children are choosy, but try making just one healthy change a day, and offer lots of variety.

606 PLAY A HEALTH TRICK

Don't feel guilty about tricking your kids into eating and drinking more healthily – it's for their own good. If they make a fuss about drinking light drinks, for example, decant sugar-free versions of their favourite fruit squashes into the usual bottles when they're not looking!

607 A CHOCOLATE DIP

Make your children a healthy but 'naughty' dessert by dipping bits of fresh fruit in melted dark chocolate and allowing it to cool, or even invest in a chocolate fondue set and get the whole family dipping. Try tropical fruits like mango and pineapple.

608 CUT SOME FAT

Cut the amounts of saturated fat in your children's sandwiches by using less butter, spread or mayonnaise and choosing low-fat fillings such as lean ham, turkey, chicken, tuna in brine, or cottage cheese.

609 SECRET INGREDIENTS

To get your family eating more vegetables without them noticing, slip them into favourite dishes – for example, add finely sliced mushrooms to Bolognese, chopped red pepper to tomato sauces and steamed leeks or celeriac to mashed potato.

610 DON'T DEPRIVE THEM

Encourage your child to eat healthily 90% of the time and let them choose and plan what they would like to eat for their 'fun foods' for the other 10% (1 or 2 snacks each day). This removes the feeling of being deprived of certain foods and wanting them even more. And because you're allowing everything in moderation, it teaches responsible food planning and fosters a sense of independence.

611 GROWING UP

As kids approach school age, they should gradually move towards a diet that's lower in fat and higher in fibre than when they were calorie-hungry youngsters. And by the age of five, their diet should mirror an adult's – low in fat, sugar and salt and high in fibre, with five portions of fruit and veg a day (see www.5aday.nhs.uk).

612 TREAT YOUR KIDS DIFFERENTLY

Remember that nutrition guidelines for adults are inappropriate for most children under the age of five. Children have small stomachs so it's important to maximize the calories in their food by, for instance, using whole milk and carbohydrate-heavy meals. They require small but frequent meals to meet their energy needs.

613 USE YOUR LOAF

Instead of biscuits and cakes, give your children healthier versions with less refined sugar like banana bread, cheese scones or fruit loaf, which have a 'cakey' taste without being too high in sugar or fat.

614 A SINGLE CHANGE

Many people go into automatic-pilot mode when cooking their usual family recipes because they cook them so often. Before you start to cook, think of one change you could implement to make it healthier – frying mushrooms in olive oil instead of butter, for example, or swapping half the meat for beans or lentils.

615 STICK TO WHAT THEY LIKE

If your children love one or two types of vegetable but won't eat the rest, don't worry. Feed them two portions of the one they like – although a varied diet is best, getting enough portions is more important. Introduce new kinds gradually.

616 STAY AT 150

If you want to let your kids have snacks but don't know how much is too much, watch the portions and keep each item around 150 calories each. In fact, make your life easier and go for pre-portioned snacks like 100-calorie packs, fun-size chocolate bars, or 25 g (1 oz) bags of crisps (potato chips).

617 THE BEST START

Children who eat a healthy diet balanced between the four main food groups – meat and fish, dairy products, fruit and vegetables, and bread, potatoes and other carbs – are much less likely to be obese or overweight as adults or to suffer from health problems such as heart disease.

618 SNACKS ON THE GO

Great ideas for kids travel snacks are chopped or sliced raw vegetables such as carrots and celery, and crackers, oat biscuits or wholewheat breads, which are full of wholegrains and low in fat and sugar.

619 DON'T FORBID FOODS

Studies have shown that forbidding foods will only make your children want them more. Help them to maintain a healthy attitude to food by allowing everything in moderation and offering healthy snacks.

620 PACK IN THE FRUIT

Try to make it a rule to put two pieces of fruit into every packed lunch you make. You don't have to stick to apples and bananas – try grapes, fruit salad, a slice of melon or a mix of dried fruit.

621 CHUNKY CHIPS

Why not swap chips (fries) for healthy homemade potato wedges? Simply cut potatoes (in their skins for added fibre) into wedges, brush with a little olive oil and bake in the oven until they are soft in the middle and crispy on the outside.

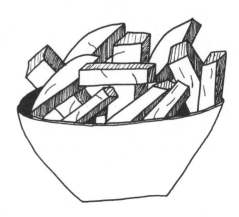

622 BE PREPARED

If you find cooking on weekdays a struggle, prepare in advance by spending an evening or afternoon at the weekend cooking up in bulk and freezing meals to ensure your family have fresh-cooked food every night.

623 FATTEN THEM UP

Children under five years old need more fat than older children and adults, but steer clear of cakes, biscuit and chocolate in favour of foods that contain plenty of other nutrients like meat, oily fish and whole dairy produce.

624 ORANGE LOVER

Oranges are high in vitamin C and they're a really good portable fruit because they don't bruise easily. Slip one into your child's lunchbox or satchel for a healthy snack.

625 FEED LITTLE MINDS

Blood-sugar levels are linked to concentration, so allowing your children to skip meals or snack on high-sugar snacks rather than low-GI alternatives (like oats and fruit) could have an effect on how well they do at school.

626 LIMIT THEIR FIBRE

Although vegetables and fruit are healthy for adults, young children shouldn't eat too many fibre-rich foods. They may fill them up so much that they can't eat enough fat and protein with them to provide adequate calories and nutrients.

627 A GOURMET BABY

Give your baby a head start in the taste stakes by puréeing and freezing unusual combinations of fruit and vegetables in ice cube trays. If you aren't sure which flavours to combine, scour the baby aisles at your local supermarket for ideas. Carrots and apples are a good starting point.

628 FRUITS OF THEIR LABOUR

Cook meals with your children and make it fun. They're more likely to eat what they've helped prepare, especially if you've given them some choice about flavours. They'll also take great pride in watching you eat what they've prepared. Also, encourage them to enjoy their food and take time to eat rather than wolfing it down.

628 TEENS IN A FIZZ

Fizzy cans of drink are unhealthy for everyone but they're particularly bad for teenage girls as they have been linked to low bone density (because they rob bones of strengthening calcium), which can cause osteoporosis. Try sparkling water instead.

630 BE PREPARED

Always have kid-friendly veggies prepared – such as baby carrots, sugar snap peas, red peppers, cherry tomatoes and washed, chopped cucumber. When your child complains he's starving between meals, you can offer him a healthy snack. If he's really hungry, he'll eat it.

631 HIDE THE TREATS

Keep chocolate, crisps (potato chips) and other unhealthy snacks in a high cupboard away from other foods. Your kids will be much more likely to demand snack foods if they can see them or they're in accessible cupboards or drawers. It's good for you too, as you may reconsider going to the trouble of reaching for the snacks.

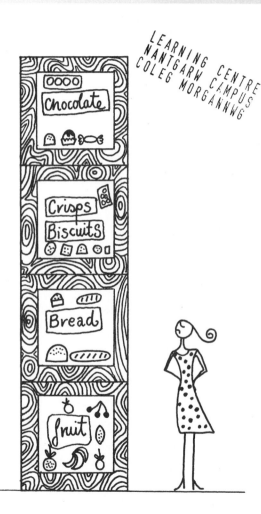

LEARNING CENTRE
NANTGARW CAMPUS
COLEG MORGANNWG

choosing fruit

632 RIPE STRAWBERRIES ONLY

With strawberries, pick only the cartons with the reddest, plumpest berries. Strawberries that are showing patches of green or white are not yet ripe and once strawberries are picked, they will not continue to ripen – if they're unripe, they'll stay that way!

633 A TRUE BLUE

Select cartons of blueberries that are wholly blue. Blueberries with a reddish tone will taste overly tart, and those that are too purple are probably overripe and will be too soft and low on taste. They're called blueberries for a reason!

634 POP YOUR CHERRY

Cherries should be firm to the touch, not squashy, and should be a uniform red or scarlet in colour with no brown patches. Those which have been in storage too long develop bruising, which means they're not as good for you.

635 AN APPLE A DAY

When you're choosing apples, go for the crispest, hardest, most blemish-free fruit you can find. Any wrinkling of the skin means the apple is too old. The skin should hold firm against your finger with no bruising. This is particularly important for Braeburn, Granny Smith and Pink Lady varieties.

636 SMELL YOUR BERRIES

The best way to check if berries are fresh is to smell them. They should smell fresh and fruity. If you're buying in cartons, make sure the carton is still dry and that no juices are in the bottom. Store them on kitchen paper towels in the fridge.

637 PLUMP IS BEAUTIFUL

With peaches, nectarines and plums, plumpness is key. The more plump and full the fruit feels, the juicier it will be. If you apply pressure on the skin of the fruit, the fruit should give way a little. If you have bought them unripe, leave them in a loosely closed brown paper bag for a day or so at room temperature to ripen.

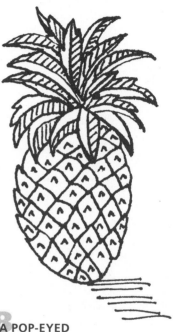

638 GET A POP-EYED PINEAPPLE

When you're choosing pineapples, look for a bright colour, a small, compact crown with bright green leaves and protruding eyes. Also, the pineapple should smell sweet and fragrant – like most fruit, if it doesn't smell it isn't usually ripe.

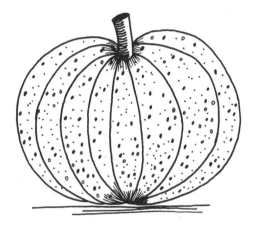

639 PUMPKIN HEAVY

Pumpkins are a great source of vitamins and betacarotene, especially in the autumn (fall). Make sure you choose those that are plump and heavy for their size with a clean, firm rind with no cracks or bruises. Those that are too light may have been in storage for too long.

640 GO MAN-GO

Mango is packed with vitamin C. When buying, don't worry if the mango is almost all green or red, as colour doesn't make any difference to how ripe it is – it's simply down to a difference in varieties. Put a little pressure on the fruit and if the flesh gives way a little bit, the mango is ripe.

641 SMELL MELONS

Cantaloupes are the easiest of the melons to judge for ripeness as they give off an aroma that's hard to miss when they're ready for eating. Always look for the most symmetrical melon and if you buy a not-quite-ripe cantaloupe, let it sit out and ripen at room temperature for a few days.

642 PICK A PAPAYA

It's hard to go wrong with papayas, but be sure to pick one that has changed from its original, unripe green to a richer yellowish or orangey colour, particularly around the larger end of the fruit.

643 BERRY GOOD

Choose raspberries that have a rich berry scent. Raspberries that still have green stems on them are not ripe. They can be expensive, so it's even more important to be discriminating.

644 CANNED TYPES

If you're buying fruit in cans, it's healthier to choose fruit preserved in its own juice, or in other fruit juices, than syrups. Syrups are high in sugar and contain more calories.

645 SQUEEZE YOUR AVOCADOS

For immediate use, select slightly soft avocados that yield to gentle pressure on the skin. For use in 4–5 days, buy firm fruits that do not yield to the squeeze test and leave them at room temperature to ripen.

646 RIPE WITH WRINKLES

Unlike most fruits, passion fruit is best when the skin sags and is wrinkly. Those with smoother skins will be too sour to use for anything but cooking. They should still feel dense, though, as those that are too light could be overripe.

647 GET HEAVY

Select watermelon that has few bruises or cuts to the flesh. A good watermelon is dense with water, so a smaller watermelon that is heavier than a larger-sized one will be a better choice. Make sure the watermelon has a slightly yellow belly, meaning it was sun-ripened, and a hollow sound if you knock on the rind.

648 BE FIRM

Tomatoes are an excellent source of vitamins and cancer-fighting antioxidants. Look for smooth-skinned, firm fruits with uniform colour. They should be firm rather than soft, and shouldn't have scarring on the skin surface – this can indicate sun damage that can reduce nutrient quality.

648 SHAKE YOUR GRAPES

The best way to pick the freshest grapes
in your supermarket is to hold a bunch
by the stem and shake them gently. If the
grapes drop off the stem they have been in
storage for too long. The ideal bunch is one
where most of the grapes are plump, clear
and firmly attached.

650 A TASTE OF HONEY

Look for honeydew melon with a yellowish-
white to creamy rind colour, with a little
bit of spotting on the rind and no cracks
or bruises. Honeydew that feels sticky to
the touch is ripe and ready, and if the skin
is giving off a faint, pleasantly sweet scent,
it's ready for eating.

651 RATTLE AND HOLD

It might make you look odd in the
supermarket aisles, but there are two
ways to check if a melon is fresh – for the
perfect ripeness, all (except watermelon)
should smell sweet at the stem end and
you shouldn't hear the seeds rattling inside
when you shake them.

652 AVOCADOS TO AVOID

Don't worry about the irregular light-brown
markings that are sometimes found on the
skin of avocados – these generally have
no effect on the flesh inside. But avoid
those with dark sunken spots or cracked or
broken surfaces as these are signs of decay.
Slow down ripening by refrigerating.

653 GREEN SKIN

Nectarines shouldn't have any green tinges
to their skin, because green patches are
unlikely to come up to ripeness before the
rest goes bad. If you have green nectarines,
why not turn them into a delicious dessert
– split in half and roast in a low oven, then
drizzle with maple syrup or natural yogurt.

654 SAY NO TO MOULD

Don't buy strawberries with any trace of
mould on them, because it spreads fast
between berries even if stored correctly.
The freshest, healthiest strawberries don't
lose their hairs when touched or washed
and are red in colour and firm. Avoid those
with large uncoloured or seeded areas.

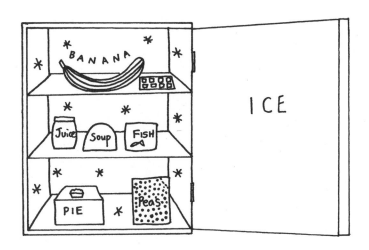

655 DON'T BIN THE BANANAS

Don't throw away overripe bananas. Use them in cooking (for banana cake or loaf) or for smoothies with other fruits or yogurt. You can also freeze them and use as an alternative to fruit sorbet or ice cream (overripe bananas freeze better than ripe ones).

656 A HARD STEM

In general, ripe melons smell pleasant and fruity when they are ready to eat. The stem end should be indented and a little soft. If the stem looks hard or withered, the melon has been in storage for too long and won't taste fresh.

657 GET HEAVY HANDED

If you're looking for the freshest citrus produce, go for those that feel heaviest. Fruits that feel light are likely to have been hanging around too long and may have started to lose their juice.

658 BERRY FRESH

Berries are a great way to give yourself a vitamin and antioxidant boost, but it's important to get them as fresh as possible. Visit farm shops or pick-your-own farms for the freshest, straight off the plant.

659 A GOOD APRICOT

Apricots should be uniform in colour, which shows they have been harvested at the right time and are fully ripe. Store at room temperature to further ripen, or in the fridge if they are already soft enough.

660 FLICK THE STALK

To test whether an avocado is ripe, flick off the small stalk at the end – if it comes off easily, the fruit is ripe. If there's no stalk, use a light squeeze instead to test for ripeness.

661 DON'T BE A SOFTIE

Don't choose melons that are too soft because they will continue to ripen and the very soft patches will go bad before long. Choose them when they are a little bit harder if you want to wait before eating.

662 CHERRY RIPE

There are many different varieties of cherries. Sweeter varieties (for eating) should have a stem and be firm to the touch. When choosing sour cherries for cooking, the stem should pop off easily when pulled.

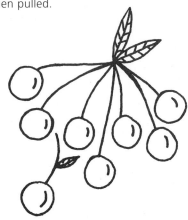

663 FIRM PLUMS

Plums taste best when they're not too soft – there should be some firmness to the skin when pressed with the flat of your thumb or finger, so the flesh springs back from the touch. Avoid relatively hard or shrivelled fruit.

664 RIPE FOR THE PICKING

Make sure you choose the ripest fruit, if possible those which have matured on trees as plant-ripened fruit have the most nutrients. Find this information on the label – it usually applies only to organic fruit.

choosing vegetables

665 LET US BE CRISP

Lettuce should be crisp to the touch when you buy it, and there should be no see-through patches on the leaves, or moisture. It's best to buy it in open packets or brown paper and keep well refrigerated.

666 CORN COLOUR

Contrary to popular belief, it doesn't matter if sweetcorn is yellow or white. Sweetness isn't determined by colour, which is naturally varied – it's determined by freshness, so make sure you choose a freshly picked ear.

667 CHOOSE CRISP CELERY

Choose large, firm celery stalks with a uniform shape and a clear white bottom. Avoid spindly, wilted stalks, or those that are too green, as these can have too strong a taste.

668 DARK SECRETS

Green, leafy vegetables are a great addition to any diet, but if you want to make sure you get the most goodness out of them, avoid those with wilted leaves or those that are too pale or yellowed in colour.

669 ARTFUL CHOKER CHOICE

The head of artichokes should be tightly closed and feel firm and heavy with no discolouration. Keep fresh in a brown paper bag or wrap in plastic in the fridge.

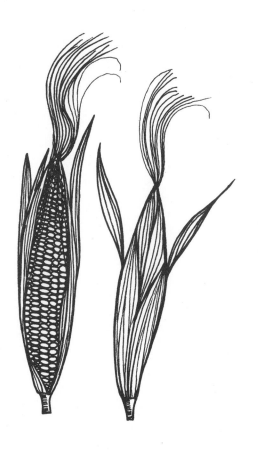

670 CHECK YOUR TASSELS

There is only one surefire way to tell if an ear of corn is fresh (and they don't stay fresh for long) and that is by the tassel at the end of it. If the tassel is soft and silky then the corn is fresh. If, on the other hand, it's starting to get hard and brittle or if it has been removed, don't buy it.

671 THE CRUNCH

For the best flavour, look for deep-orange coloured carrots with smooth-skinned roots. Fresh-looking tops mean they have been recently harvested. Avoid those with purple or green shoulders or those that are pale in colour, and steer clear of those with forked or oversized roots.

672 WASH YOUR LEEKS

For leeks to taste their best and give you the best dose of healthiness, they should have long white shanks and dark green leaf tissue. Avoid dry or yellowish leaves or discoloured shanks. And remember to wash inside the outer layers, where dirt and grit can accumulate, under cold running water.

673 FIRMNESS IS KEY

If you're choosing aubergine (or eggplant), go for firm, shiny dark purple fruit with small blossom scars. Avoid soft, bronze or green-coloured fruits or those with a dried stem, or calyx – it should be bright and green. Older aubergines tend to have a bitter or acidic taste.

674 GREEN SHOULDERS

Parsnips and turnips should have clean, smooth, firm and well-shaped roots with light, even-coloured skin. Those that are sunburned (which have green shoulders) are likely to be low on flavour and if they're soft they'll be woody.

675 CHOOSE TIGHT BUNCHES

If you want to make sure you're choosing the best broccoli, Brussels sprouts or cauliflower, choose tightly compacted flower clusters on broccoli and cauliflower, and compact, uniform sprouts. Avoid wilted, yellow, or dirty heads, and avoid loose, open sprouts or those that are yellow or pale green.

676 AVOID ARTICHOKE FLOWERS

If you're hunting for the perfect artichoke look for tight, solid buds on fruits that are heavy for their size. Avoid ones with loose buds or purple flowers forming, which are overmature. If they're fresh, they'll be squeaky when rubbed against each other.

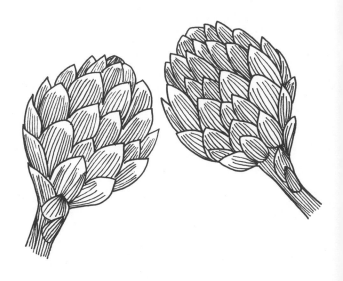

677 GO GREEN WITH ASPARAGUS

Asparagus should be mostly green in colour (those with white colouring are invariably less tender, even when fresh) and choose firm stalks with close, compact tips. The sooner it's used the more tender it will be, but don't forget to cut off the woody white end before cooking.

678 SNAP A SUGAR SNAP

Avoid sugar snap peas with dry-looking, rusty, wilted or damaged pods, as they might have been hanging around for a while. Pods should be plump, uniform in colour and crisp – reject them if you can see large seeds through the skin, which means they will have lost their freshness.

679 GET WITH THE BEET

For beetroot, the key to flavour is in appearance – look for smooth round uniform bunches with small to medium roots. Avoid beetroots that are blocky or angular in shape, rough-skinned or oversized. Freshness of tops or leaves is not an indication of quality.

680 DON'T SUPERSIZE YOUR RADISHES

Choose radishes with medium-sized firm crisp roots. Avoid wilted or soft roots, which is a sign of them being too old, or oversized roots, which will taste pithy. And choose smoother skins, because those with growth cracks retain fewer nutrients.

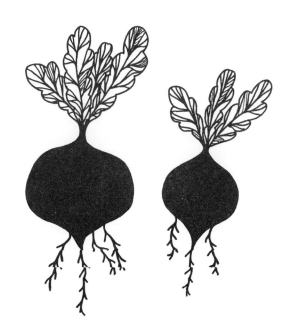

681 PEPPER SPOT

For the healthiest addition to your lunchtime salad, choose peppers that have a uniform colour. Those that have contrasting colour spots may have had sun damage, which can reduce the nutrients and vitamins they contain.

682 COOL YOUR SPUDS

Try to buy potatoes as close to cooking them as you can, but if you have to store them for a while, keep them in a cool dark place away from sunlight and preferably in paper. Potatoes which have sprouted tubers have less flavour, and green tinges prevent them cooking well.

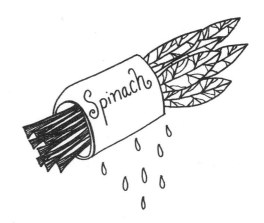

683 GARLIC HEAD

Garlic tastes best when the heads are firm and plump with no green shoots. Green shoots coming out of the bulbs means the garlic has been in storage too long and will taste less fresh and may be slightly bitter. The bulbs can still be used for cooking, although they won't taste as good, but discard the green bits.

684 HIDE THE SPINACH

Spinach contains many great nutrients and antioxidants and is a really versatile vegetable, so it's great for adding a 'hidden' vegetable kick to dishes. Spinach should have bright green leaves when it's fresh, not yellowed or dry looking, and is best kept airtight or with stalks wrapped in damp paper towels.

685 A GOOD BEET

Beetroot should be used quickly, before its sugar turns to starch, which can make it taste fluffy. It should be hard to the touch and if you're buying it with the greenery attached, make sure there's no wilting.

686 SWEET BROCCOLI

If your broccoli smells like cabbage, it's probably been hanging around too long. Broccoli should be completely green and not yellowing, and should smell sweet and fresh.

687 PACK A PUNCH

Cauliflower is freshest and healthiest when the tops are light in colour without any discoloured patches, and when the florets are tightly packed. If the stalks bend when you touch it, it's been in storage too long.

688 SPROUT A FRESH CHOICE

The best way to buy Brussels sprouts is to buy them still attached to the stalk – that way they'll keep more of their moisture. Cut or break them off the stalk just before use for maximum health benefits.

689 DON'T SPLIT YOUR PEAS

If you're buying garden peas in the pod, the pods should be whole but not split at the sides, which means they're overripe. One of the healthiest ways to buy them is frozen because peas hold a lot of their nutrients that way.

690 PICKING PARSNIPS

With parsnips, the general rule is that the fresher they are, the whiter the flesh. Try to avoid those that are yellowing or brown around the central core as these are likely to have been in storage for too long.

691 GET RID OF THE GREENS

Rhubarb, carrots and other vegetables you buy with greens attached will store better if you remove the green tops to prevent them absorbing the vegetable's water and reducing nutrient content.

buying meat & fish

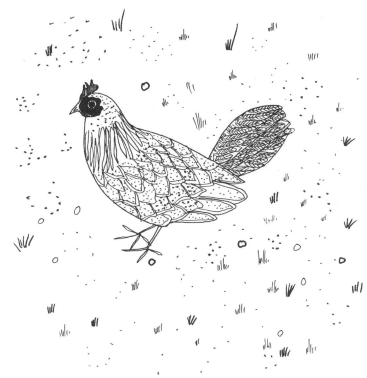

682 BUY FREE-RANGE BIRDS

Always buy free-range chickens, which will have been reared with enough space to move around freely and develop muscle tone. The meat will be leaner and better for you than the meat from less-mobile birds.

693 BEEF IT UP

When shopping for beef, choose sirloin or topside as they are the leanest cuts. Sirloin has only 3.8 g fat per 100 g serving and topside 5.2 g, compared to 24.1 g fat for minced (ground) beef. Spend the same amount of money – just buy less of the leaner, more expensive cuts.

694 LEAN CUISINE

If you're looking for meat or poultry that will last longer, go lean. Lean cuts last longer than fatty meats because it's the fat on meat that first starts to decay.

695 PIG ON PORK

Pork is often thought to be a fatty meat but it's healthy because not as much of it is saturated as with other meats – the level of fat depends entirely on which cut you choose, so go for leaner cuts like tenderloin (3.6 g fat per 100 g/3.5 oz), which has half the fat of other cuts.

696 IT'S IN THE EYES

If you're buying fresh fish whole, look at the eyes, which should be clear, and the gills, which should be transparent and bright red in colour. Don't be afraid to ask the fishmonger to show you the fish close up – they might give you a fresher fish if they think you know what you're looking for!

697 DON'T BE GREY

Lamb should never be grey or sweaty, which means it's either been hanging around too long or has been in and out of hot and cold environments too much and won't have retained its characteristic aromatic taste. The flesh should be pink and the fat white.

698 BEEF UP THE DARK

The best-tasting beef should be a dark red colour with slightly yellowish fat. If the fat is too white or the meat is bright red, the beef hasn't been hung for long enough and will be lower on taste and tougher. It's better if there's some fat marbled throughout, as this makes it more tender.

699 DON'T DITCH THE FAT

It might sound counter-intuitive, but buying fattier meat can actually help you take smaller portions, because (as long as you cut off the fat on your plate) you are likely to eat less. Also, fattier meat generally has a better taste, so it will be more satisfying.

700 PINKY AND PORKY

Pork is one of those meats which can harbour salmonella bacteria, so it's important that you buy fresh meat which has been properly stored. Look for meat that is pink and firm to the touch with very white fat. If the fat is too yellow or the meat is grey, you should reject it.

701 GET FRESH FISH

It's difficult to know how fresh fish is when it's on the rack – even if you visit a specialist fishmonger, it could be three days old if you're in the city. The best way to ensure fish is fresh is to buy really fresh in bulk from a market and freeze. Buying frozen fish can also be a good option, as it is often frozen quickly and therefore has less time to deteriorate.

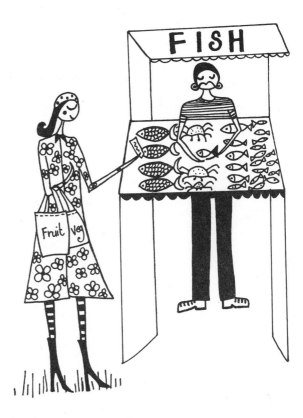

702 YOU CAN'T BEAT A BUTCHER

Most people think butchers are more
expensive than supermarkets for
buying meat, but the opposite is
often true. A good butcher will
be able to help you get the
best meat for your money,
so ask for advice.

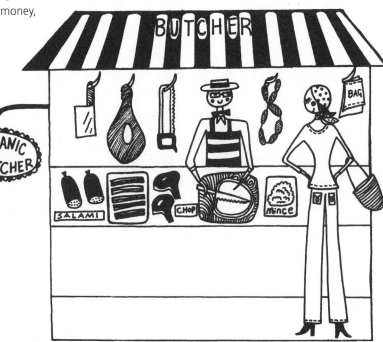

703 FISHY ISN'T DISHY

If you want to check your fish is fresh, look for light scales and a slightly slimy sheen to the skin. Fish that looks dry or where the scales are dark or peeling is too old. Above all, it shouldn't smell too 'fishy'– really fresh fish has very little odour.

704 THE RIGHT LIGHTING

If you buy your meat in a supermarket, try to examine your choice away from the brightly lit meat counters, which are often too bright for you to see the real colour of the meat. Take it to a different aisle and make your choice there.

705 DON'T BE A FARM FAN

Salmon and trout are great choices if you're eating fish because they're high in omega-3 oils and low in the damaging mercury deposits that can build up in other cold-water fish. Farmed fish, however, are lower in omega-3s and the flesh is less lean. Choose wild or organic whenever you can.

buying flavourings & condiments

706 BUY SMALL

If you don't use spices and dried herbs very often in your cooking, buy the smallest quantities you can. Ground, blended and chopped spices last around six months in your cupboard before they start to lose their potency, while whole spices can keep their taste for up to a year.

707 BE AN EXTRA VIRGIN

Labelling of olive oils can be confusing, with early and late varieties, single estates and different extraction methods. The most important label to look for is 'extra virgin', which means it's taken from the first pressing of the olives and is therefore finer in flavour and best for dressings.

708 SEND FOR THE SALSA

Instead of buying commercially prepared tomato ketchup, choose fresh salsa – or buy tomatoes, red peppers and chilli and make your own. Chop them up and mix together to make a great alternative to ketchup for meat, eggs and burgers.

buying organic

709 TWO SHOPS ARE BETTER THAN ONE

Organic fruit and vegetables often don't keep as long as non-organic so you'll have to think about how you shop as well as how you eat. It might mean two trips instead of one and making better use of your freezer.

710 TOTALLY FREE TIPPLE

If you want to be sure your wine and beer is free of pesticides it's best to choose organic. However, some health experts say it doesn't make any difference as the time the alcohol is stored for fermentation means the chemicals break down anyway.

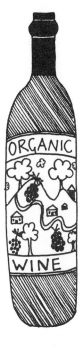
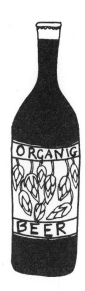

shopping tips

711 BECOME A CONVERT

Organic meat is often more expensive, especially if you buy it from supermarkets. Look for 'in conversion' labels (also labelled 'free range additive free'), which is food from farms undergoing the two-year conversion to organic status.

712 COCOA LOCO

Don't deprive yourself completely of chocolate but do choose dark organic varieties, which are high in cocoa solids. They're expensive, but so rich that a few squares is usually enough to satisfy, and they contain antioxidants so will give you a health kick, too.

713 PRIORITIZE FOR PRICE

The decision to buy organic food can be restrictive as it's often more expensive than non-organic. Solve it by converting bit by bit rather than in one go – each time you shop, bring home one more organic item so you build it up slowly. Choose meat, dairy, fruit and vegetable organics above other kinds of food to start with.

714 ON SPECIAL OFFER

Take time to compare fresh, frozen, and canned foods to see which is cheapest. Buying what's on special offer can be a great way to get cheap, healthy food and is often linked to what's in season. Many of these foods can be bought fresh and then frozen for longer-term value.

715 ORDER YOUR LIST

Before you go shopping, make a list of all the foods you need, then you won't forget anything. If you know your supermarket well, arrange your list according to where foods are placed, so you can go through the list in order as you work your way through the shop.

716 AIR-CON THE CAR

If you have air conditioning in your car, put your summer shopping on the back seat rather than in the boot, because it's likely to be cooler there, which will help food stay at the right temperature.

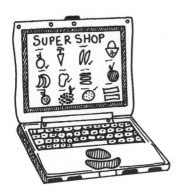

718 SHOP ONLINE

If you're short on shopping time, why not try ordering your basics on the internet? Many supermarkets and local shops now have internet ordering and delivery sites and you can make sure you're always stocked up with the basics.

720 DON'T BE FOOLED

Ready-prepared convenience foods often appear to be good value, and may even claim to be healthy choices, but they are rarely as healthy as fresh foods because they contain more fat, sugar and salt. If you must buy pre-packed and processed foods, make sure you read the nutrition labels carefully and choose those lower in fat, sodium and calories and higher in vitamins, fibre and other nutrients.

717 STORE YOUR VOUCHERS

In order not to forget those all-important money-off and discount coupons when you're doing your supermarket shop, write out your shopping list on an old envelope and put your vouchers inside.

718 STICK TO YOUR LIST

Make yourself a list before you go shopping and stick to it – that way, you won't be tempted to indulge in all those high-sugar treats the supermarkets leave by the till.

721 TWO-FOR-ONES

Don't be tempted by two-for-one or three-for-two offers on unhealthy foods as studies have shown people with more in their cupboards generally tend to eat more. Buy only as much as you need.

722 BUILD UP THE BASICS

Often, people resort to ready meals and take-aways because they just can't get to the shops. Make sure your cupboards are always stocked with the basics for producing a quick meal – such as canned or frozen vegetables, meat and fish, and dried pasta and rice.

723 CHECK OUT YOUR LOCAL

Many people don't use their local shops – which can offer really good quality and value – because they haven't got time to visit during working hours. But it's worth paying them a visit to check if they do a home-delivery scheme so you can get the best of both worlds.

724 BACK BOX SCHEMES

Instead of buying your fruit and vegetables off the supermarket shelves, where they might have been imported from all over the world, why not subscribe to a local organic fruit and vegetable box scheme? Most areas have them, where fresh foods are delivered weekly often from local farms.

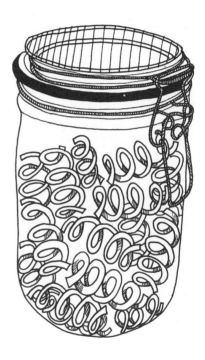

725 THE WHOLE SHOP

Remember that shopping in local healthfood and wholefood shops is a different experience to the local supermarket, and often, things aren't labelled as clearly. But don't let that put you off – the assistants expect, and are usually more than willing, to give advice.

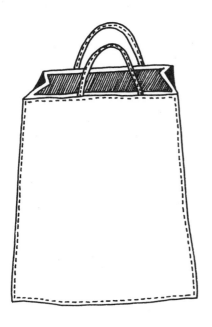

726 MAKE A COMPARISON

If you're worried about comparing how healthy foods are, it's easier to compare the fat, salt and sugar content of 100 g of the product with the same amount of another product rather than to rely on serving size, which may alter between products.

727 HONESTY IS THE BEST POLICY

If you're looking at the labels of a food to see how healthy it is, be realistic and honest about your serving size. If you always find yourself eating three biscuits, don't just look at the fat and sugar content of one. Remember to multiply!

728 GO STRAIGHT HOME

Cars heat up in the summer months, which means that your shopping heats up too if it's stored in the car for any significant length of time – not a good idea for fresh and frozen food. Solve the problem by doing your food shop last so it's not left hanging around, then head straight home. Alternatively, use your own insulated cool bags, which are useful for smaller shops.

storing your food

729 KEEP IT COOL

Keep your fridge below 40°C (104°F) if you want to make sure your food is kept as safe as possible, because eating food that has been stored in refrigerators warmer than this temperature can increase the risk of food-borne illness.

730 DON'T BE A BRUISER

Take care to avoid bruising or mashing fruits and vegetables when transporting or storing them. It doesn't just make them look bad, it also oxidizes antioxidants and destroys nutrients. And one bruised fruit or veg will cause others to become rotten or ripen much faster, so remove any that are and use them straight away.

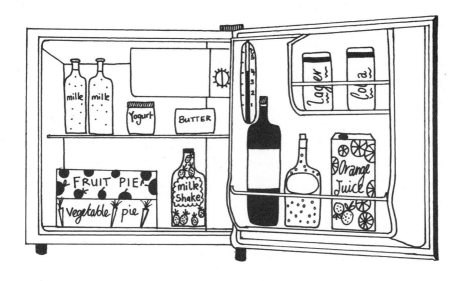

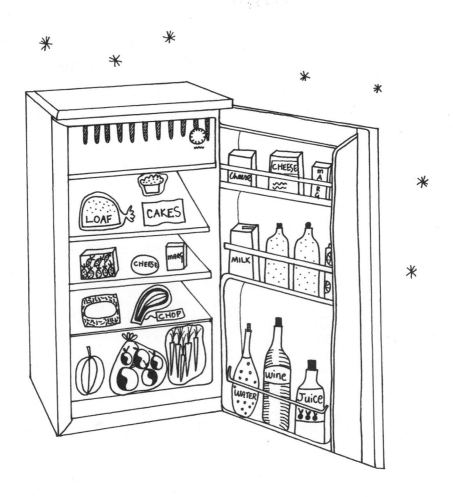

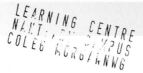

731 GET THE LOW DOWN

It's best to store raw meat and fish covered on a tray on the bottom shelf of your fridge or in the boxes at the bottom. This will make sure none of the juices escape and drip on to other foods. It is also usually marginally colder at the bottom because cold air is more dense.

732 MAKE SOME SPACE

Avoid overfilling your refrigerator – cool air must be allowed to circulate to keep food at the proper temperature wherever it's placed. Try to space food evenly throughout and avoid stacking too many items on top of each other. Most people tend to over-buy anyway, so buy less more frequently.

733 EGGS-TRA SAFE

Eggs don't have to be stored in the fridge. A cool place will do, especially as most recipes assume that the required eggs will be at room temperature. They should be stored, thin-end down, away from strong smells because the shells are porous and can absorb strong flavours.

734 SPUDS YOU LIGHT

Store your potatoes in a cool dark place. If you leave them exposed to too much light, they will turn a greenish colour. The substance that causes this to happen can be mildly toxic and therefore should not be eaten, especially by children.

735 CHECK FOR DAMAGE

Never eat any foods from jars or tins which appear damaged or look as if they might have been opened. If stored food has come into contact with air, it is likely to have been spoiled and is best returned or disposed of.

736 CUT OUT THE LIGHT

Spices and dried herbs keep their flavour better if stored in a cupboard away from heat, light and moisture, all of which impair flavour, change colour and shorten life. Try attaching a spice rack to the inside of your cupboard door. As a general rule, herbs and ground spices will retain their best flavour for a year. Whole spices can last for up to one year.

737 KEEP DRY DRY

Store all your dry foods like flour and pasta on one dry shelf, and make it a higher shelf than for wetter ingredients such as oils and vinegars. This way, the humidity levels will be just right for keeping foods at their best for longer.

739 DON'T CLING TO PLASTICS

Clingfilm (plastic wrap) contains plasticizers which are said to leach into food. Use paper, foil or reusable sealed containers, especially for high-fat foods like cheese which are highly absorbent. Or choose food wrap which is made without toxins.

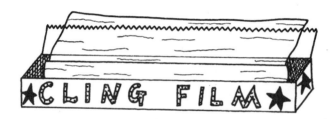

738 HUMIDITY CHECK

The cupboard under your sink can be more humid than other cupboards because of the water going through the pipes. Remember this when you're considering storage, as fruit and vegetables rot quicker in humid environments.

740 BE A HONEY

If you're looking for the ultimate food to keep in your cupboards for years, choose good old-fashioned honey, which is the only food that doesn't spoil. In fact, archaeologists have even found edible honey in the tombs of Pharaohs!

741 TOO COLD FOR COMFORT

Potatoes will actually keep for longer outside the refrigerator as being too cold causes the starch in them to turn to sugar. A cool, dry, dark place is best.

742 KEEP CHEMICALS CLEAR

Don't store foods near household cleaning products and chemicals. It's unlikely, but possible that chemicals could leach into foods, especially if the foods are to be eaten raw or if they're absorbent, like dairy products and vegetables.

743 SEPARATE DRAWERS

Store fruits and vegetables in separate drawers in your fridge. Even when chilled, fruits give off ethylene gas that shortens the shelf life of other fruit and vegetables by causing them to ripen more quickly.

744 SUN SENSITIVE

Light is the enemy of oil! Buy olive oil in dark glass bottles and keep it in a cool dark place to preserve quality. Sunlight can oxidize the oil, turning it rancid.

745 LOOK FOR STORAGE ADVICE

Always check the labels on cans or jars to determine how the contents should be stored. If you've neglected to refrigerate items that should be kept cold, it's usually best to throw them out.

extending shelf life

746 CLEAR CUCUMBERS

If you're storing cucumber in your fridge and want it to stay fresh, keep it away from apples and tomatoes, which will shorten its life. Cucumber stays fresh for up to a week, then the water content starts to drop.

747 KEEP YOUR ONIONS

Yellow and brown onions keep for longer than red onions because they have a lower sugar content. Store in an open space that's cool and dry, away from bright light, which can make them bitter. Don't store under the sink or anywhere that may be damp.

748 A GOOD EGG

Eggs should keep for around four to five weeks if they are kept refrigerated. However, bear in mind they might have been two weeks old when you first bought them, so keep an eye on the 'best before' date. Always store with the pointed side down – this keeps the yolk in the centre and helps to keep them fresh.

749 APPLE YOUR SUGAR

If brown sugar becomes solid, add a slice of apple to the container for a couple of days to restore the moisture and the balance. And keep it soft by storing a few marshmallows in the bag.

750 BURIED GINGER

If you want to keep ginger fresh for adding a healthy zing to smoothies, soups and casseroles, as well as aiding digestion, follow the ancient Chinese method of storing it – fill a small clay pot with white sand or sandy potting soil and bury the ginger root inside – it will keep for months and will also start to grow.

751 PAIR UP POTATOES

If you want to store potatoes without them budding, put an apple into the bag with them. It will help them stay smooth and eye-free for longer in your cupboard.

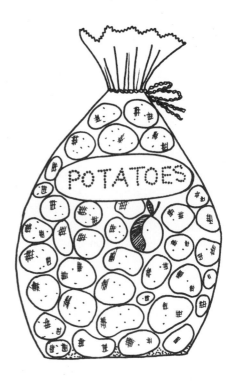

752 BAKING SODA FRESHNESS

Many people have a cupboard full of baking ingredients they don't have time to use regularly – baking soda, for example. Check if your baking soda is still fresh by pouring half a teaspoon of lemon juice or vinegar over a small pile of it. If it bubbles, it's still fresh enough to use.

753 FRESH SARNIES

To keep sandwiches fresh right through the day (or night, if you prepare them the evening before) wrap them in a piece of kitchen towel before packing them in a sealed box or bag. The paper will soak up excess moisture, leaving the sandwich soft and fresh.

754 MUD IS GOOD

If you buy organic vegetables that are still muddy, don't wash them before putting them in the fridge or larder. The mud acts as a natural preservative, preventing light from reaching the surface of the veg and helping to keep it cool. They might not look pretty, but they taste just as good.

755 DE-HUMIDIFY YOUR VEG

Line vegetable drawers in the fridge with a section of newspaper wrapped in kitchen towel. This will act as a de-humidifier, soaking up the excess moisture that can cause vegetables to rot or go mouldy.

756 RICE ON TOAST

Rice will keep in the fridge for longer if you store a slice of toast on top of it. The toast will absorb excess moisture and keep the rice fluffy and fresh.

757 DON'T SHAKE OR STIR

If you like your yogurt thick and creamy, don't stir it. Stirring changes the consistency and makes it more runny – perfect if you're using it instead of single cream, but not if you want a healthy dollop.

758 BETTER APART

If you want your potatoes to last longer, don't store them near onions, even if you're refrigerating them. Being in close proximity to onions can cause potatoes to rot more quickly.

759 DON'T TOUCH THE WALLS

Take care that delicate salad items such as cucumber and lettuce don't touch the walls of your fridge, where the high moisture content and low temperatures can cause them to go off more quickly. Keep them in the centre of shelves.

760 SUGAR YOUR CHEESE

Cheese can go off pretty quickly, developing mould within a week even if stored in the fridge – and tempting you to eat it up quickly! Prolong its life and help keep it mould-free by adding a couple of sugar cubes to your cheese containers.

761 KEEP TABS ON THE FRIDGE

To keep the contents of your fridge healthy, don't crowd the refrigerator or freezer so that you can't see what's on the shelves and air can't circulate. Check the leftovers in covered dishes and storage bags daily for spoilage. Anything that looks or smells suspicious should be thrown out.

762 BLANCH BEFORE STORAGE

To keep all the goodness and vitamin content of your vegetables, blanch them before storing – blanching kills the enzymes that cause rotting. Plunge into boiling water then straight into cold water to refresh. Cook up quickly when you need them.

763 FRUIT AT THE FRONT

Be honest, how many times have you bought healthy fruit and stored it in the fridge, only to forget all about it and find it a few weeks later, rotting at the back? Store fruit on its own shelf or at the front of the fridge to remind you it's there.

764 KEEP A TIGHT LID ON IT

The best way to store biscuits or other foods that you want to keep really dry is in jars with screw top lids, or press-top storage jars that keep the air out more effectively than other lids. Tins don't generally tend to be airtight once they've been used for a few months.

765 STEER CLEAR OF THE DOOR

Don't put eggs or milk in the refrigerator door because the temperature fluctuates more there, and you need to keep dairy products really cold to ensure they stay fresh for longer. Place them on a shelf in their original carton, which helps them retain moisture.

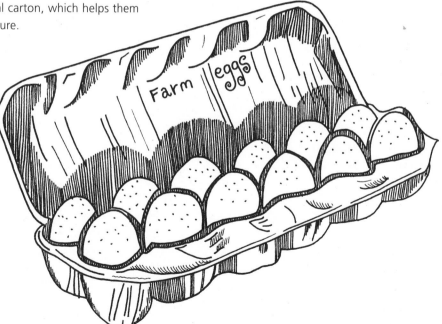

766 KEEP YEAST COOL

If you use a bread maker or make your own breads, store yeast in the fridge where it keeps for much longer and in much better condition than in your cupboard. Old yeast can reduce the bread's rising significantly.

767 COOKIE REVIVAL

If you don't want to throw out biscuits just because they've become hard, place them in a sandwich bag with a piece of bread overnight and the next day you'll have soft cookies again – but it only works once.

768 IT'S A WRAP

Store flour in a cool, dry, well-ventilated place. Keep it in the bag and wrap it in another plastic bag to prevent it from being attacked by weevils and stay fresh.

769 ZAP YOUR BERRIES

If you find yourself with a leftover bowl of strawberries you don't want to waste, liquidize them with a little sugar and freeze. Use as a healthy sorbet or compôte instead of ice cream.

770 GINGER PRESERVE

Keep ginger root for a long time in your fridge by immersing it in alcohol, which will preserve it. Sherry and vodka work well, and when it's finished you've got ginger-flavoured liquids to add to cooking as well.

keeping things fresh

771 PILLOW TALK

Don't throw away an old pillowcase – it makes an excellent lettuce bag to keep leafy greens fresh and crisp in the fridge. Wash and dry them thoroughly, then hang the pillowcase in your fridge.

772 LEFTOVER FLESH

As a guideline, cover and refrigerate leftover fish and meat within two hours of serving. Fish should be eaten within two days, and meat within three, after being taken off the bone.

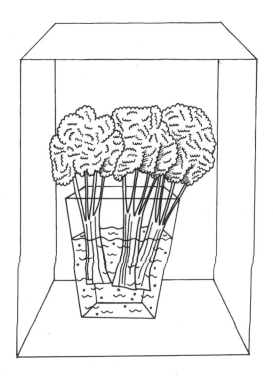

773 A BUNCH OF BROCCOLI

Broccoli will keep for a couple of weeks if you store it like a bouquet of flowers in the fridge – cut about an inch off the stem and submerge the stem in a bowl or tub of water. Change the water every couple of days and if the base of the stem seems a little slimy, snip the ends off. Broccoli can also be kept in a plastic bag.

774 TOFU TIPS

Once you have opened a package of tofu, you should store the unused portion in a container of water, with a tight-fitting lid. Tofu should be used within three days from when you first open the package and the water should be changed daily.

775 THE OTHER HALF

If you've used half an aubergine (eggplant) and want to keep the other half fresh, put it in a sealed plastic bag in the fridge and rub the cut side with lemon juice to stop it going brown. Make sure it's kept airtight and it should stay fresh for a couple of days.

776 KEEP MILK COOL

Full milk will stay fresh for 24 days if kept cold but it is very sensitive to temperature and goes off quickly. You will reduce its shelf life drastically by leaving it out for just two hours, so get into the habit of putting your milk back in the fridge as soon as you've finished with it.

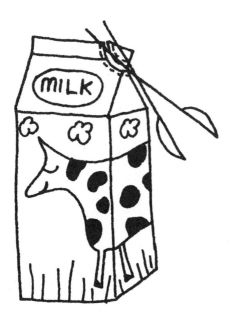

777 ENHANCE TOMATO FLAVOUR

To bring out the most flavour in tomatoes, store them in a basket on your work surface as chilling them below 55°C (130°F) can harm the flavour. They don't keep as long out of the fridge, so if you're going to do this it's best to buy them no more than one or two days before use.

778 MELLOW YELLOW

For unripe fruit you want to soften up in a hurry, leave at room temperature in a bowl with a couple of ripe bananas, which give off enzymes that help other fruit to ripen quicker. Conversely, if you want fruit to ripen slowly keep your bananas in a separate bowl.

779 PAY ATTENTION, HONEY

If honey becomes crystallized in the jar, it doesn't mean it's gone off – it just needs a little attention. Just warm the jar up gently in a microwave (be careful of metallic labels and lids) or put in a pan of hot water for a few minutes. A quick stir and it will be as good as new.

780 KEEP FLAVOUR IN PAPER

To get the most out of your mushrooms and aubergines, store them in paper bags in the fridge and only wash or wipe them just before use, which will keep them drier for longer and help them retain more flavour.

781 COOKING WITH YOGURT

Preserve the benefits of the active cultures in your yogurt by not heating it above 50°C (120°F). High temperatures can kill the beneficial bacteria in yogurts so if you want to use it in cooking, try adding it at the end.

782 THE YOLK'S ON ME

If you have a recipe that uses egg whites, you can refrigerate the yolks for later use by storing them, unbroken, in a small bowl, covered with cold water for up to two days.

783 UNDER WRAPS

Always cover your butter, as it is a very absorbent substance that will absorb fridge odours, making it taste or smell funny. The last thing you want is breakfast toast tinged with last night's curry or garlicky sauce!

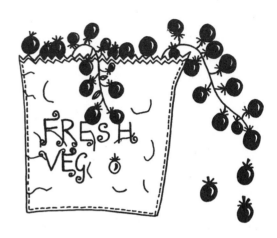

784 BAG A RIPE ONE

To speed up the process of ripening tomatoes, keep them in a brown paper bag or closed container to trap the ethylene gas that helps them ripen. Adding an ethylene-emitting apple or pear can also help.

785 UPSIDE DOWN IT

Sour cream will keep longer in your fridge if you store the container upside down, which reduces the amount of oxidizing air that can find its way into the package. Be careful when you open it, though!

786 NOT TOO RIPE

Apples are one of the few fruits which are best eaten slightly underripe, when they are still crunchy. If you keep your apples in the fridge, the cold air will slow down the ripening process but not stop it completely, It's best to buy just a few at a time to maximize your eating pleasure!.

787 PICK PAPER

Try to avoid food packaged in plastic as much as possible if the food is absorbent, such as meats and cheeses, which could take up toxins from the plastic. Choose paper packages instead, or buy fresh and remove packaging when you get home.

788 FREEZE YOUR LOAF

Bread goes stale faster in the fridge than on the counter. Freezing, however, is an excellent way to keep it fresh if you cannot finish it in one day. Cut bread, bagels and buns before freezing, then toast to defrost. Make sure the bread is protected from freezer burn by closing the bag tightly.

789 FOIL YOUR CELERY

To keep your celery fresh and crisp in the fridge for weeks, wrap it completely in aluminium foil to keep the moisture in.

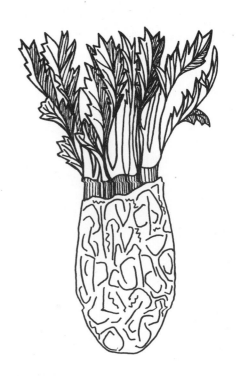

780 GRAPE FULL

Store your grapes in the coldest part of the fridge in a plastic bag. Make sure you wash them well before you serve them to avoid pesticide residues and other toxins, but don't wash them before you refrigerate as this can cause them to rot.

781 REMOVE MOULD

While not a major health threat, mould can make food unappetizing. Don't eat the mould or food that has come into contact with it. Hard cheeses, salami and firm fruits and vegetables can be saved from mould if you cut out the mould and also a large area around it, where there might be growth beneath the surface of the food.

782 WASH AND SERVE

Don't prepare your strawberries and raspberries too early if you want them to stay fresh – you can hull or slice them earlier, but only wash them just before you serve, then pat dry with kitchen towel to help them keep their fresh texture.

783 PAPER MUSHROOMS

When you bring fresh mushrooms home from shopping, remove them from any plastic wrapping and put them into a paper bag. Fold the top closed and the mushrooms will last a week.

784 AVOID THE PLASTIC FANTASTIC

Don't keep meat in plastic in your fridge unless you're going to eat it the same day. Instead, put it on a plate covered with kitchen roll or a tea towel so the meat can breathe but is protected.

785 BLEACH WITH LEMONS

Lemon juice is a great way to stop pre-sliced fruit turning brown and unappetizing, and it will give it a fruitier, more intense taste too. Use it on apples, pears and bananas.

786 DON'T COVER STRAWBERRIES

The moisture content of fresh strawberries is high, so store uncovered or loosely covered – covering the berries up can cause them to rot, even when refrigerated.

797 LEAVE SEEDS ATTACHED

When using only part of a red, green or yellow (bell) pepper, cut it from the bottom or the sides, leaving the seeds attached, and it will remain moist for longer. You can put the rest in a resealable plastic bag and use it 3–4 days later.

798 FISH FOR SAFETY

Seafood is responsible for a lot of food poisoning, but it's perfectly safe and very healthy if treated correctly. If you can't use it immediately, remove it from its original wrapping and rinse in cold water. Wrap loosely in plastic wrap, store in the coldest part of the refrigerator, and use within 2 days. Store ready-to-eat fish such as smoked mackerel separately from raw fish.

799 FOOD POISONING

Although you might be tempted to keep foods in your fridge and cupboards for a long time, there are certain foods which you should never keep more than a few days – most importantly fresh or thawed meat and fish, and cooked rice.

800 A QUICK REFRESH

If your lettuce is looking a little droopy, try a restaurant trick by refreshing it before you serve it. Fill a bowl with ice cubes and water and plunge the lettuce into it to give it back a bit of its lost crispness.

801 KEEP LETTUCE DRY

To keep lettuce fresher longer wrap a dry paper towel around the root end of the lettuce head and store in a freezer bag or in a sealed plastic container in your fridge. The paper towel will absorb the excess water.

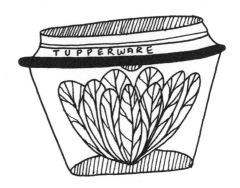

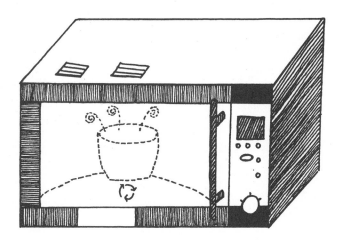

freezing & reheating

802 MEAT-FREEZE ZONE

If you want to freeze raw meat at home, make sure you do it before the 'use by' date, and preferably as soon as you get it home. Defrost properly, try to use within one day of defrosting and make sure it's cooked right through before serving.

803 USE THE RIGHT SETTING

If you're defrosting meat or fish in the microwave, choose the defrost setting or use low power to stop the outer edges of the food cooking before the middle defrosts. Arrange loose pieces of fish or meat in a single layer with thickest parts or largest pieces towards the outside.

804 CAN'T FREEZE EVERYTHING

You can freeze any food except canned or preserved food or whole eggs. Some foods, however, do not freeze well. High-fat dairy products like cream and mayonnaise tend to separate when defrosted, and high-water content vegetables such as lettuce and cucumber will go soggy.

805 THE BIG FREEZE

The freezer should be below -18°C (0°F). If items are not frozen solid, then the temperature is too low. Check from time to time and throw food away the minute you notice any slight defrosting, because harmful bacteria could be thriving in the too-warm conditions.

806 DON'T DOUBLE YOUR JEOPARDY

You can refreeze frozen food that has partially thawed as long as it still contains frozen areas. If it has thawed through, however, or has been at room temperature rather than refrigerated, you shouldn't refreeze it and it should either be cooked or discarded.

807 WARM UP SLOWLY

It is not ideal to defrost food at room temperature. The best way to defrost is by planning ahead and allowing the food to defrost slowly in the fridge. If you're not organized enough to do this, use the microwave. But as it can partially cook food, it's best to cook the food directly after defrosting as it is not safe to keep partially cooked food in the fridge.

808 COOK IT THROUGH

Contrary to popular belief, freezing doesn't actually kill bacteria or other food microbes, but what it does do is put them in a dormant state so they won't be active or reproducing until the food is thawed again. This is why it's important to cook food thoroughly after defrosting.

809 ICE IN SOME FLAVOUR

Don't worry that freezing your meals will harm them or lessen the flavour – in fact, for dishes such as lasagne and stews freezing can be beneficial as it increases the diffusion of antioxidant-rich herbs and spices.

810 TAKE A BATH

If you don't want to use the microwave – or you're defrosting something too big to fit in – you can submerge the food in cold water, remembering to change the water every 30 minutes to speed up the thawing process. Certain types of food can become watery with this method, but it's great for joints of meat and poultry.

811 FREEZE YOUR EGGS

The best way to make sure you don't waste eggs, especially if you cook or bake a lot, is to separate the eggs and freeze whites and yolks separately in a lightly oiled ice-cube tray. When frozen, pop them out and store in separate ziplock bags in the freezer.

812 GET A THERMOMETER

Don't just rely on your inbuilt thermometer to ensure that your fridge is at the right temperature. Invest in an appliance thermometer and check regularly that your refrigerator is at 4°C (40°F) or colder and your freezer is at -18°C (0°F).

813 THAW IT COLD

Thaw meat in the refrigerator rather than on your kitchen surface, where food is more susceptible to bacteria and might thaw too quickly. Store meat and fish on a dish on the bottom shelf as they defrost, so that the juices don't drip on to other foods and contaminate them.

814 TURN UP THE HEAT

If you're using leftovers, make sure they are piping hot throughout when reheating, to ensure that any bacteria or microbes are killed off – bacteria are destroyed very quickly with heat. Gravies and soups should be heated to a rolling boil, and other food to 74°C (165°F). Refrigerated leftovers should be used within 3 days.

815 CRUMBS!

If you have unused digestive biscuits (graham crackers) in your cupboard, crush them up and add melted butter to make a cheesecake base, then freeze. Simply mix together cream cheese, condensed milk and lemon juice to make a quick topping.

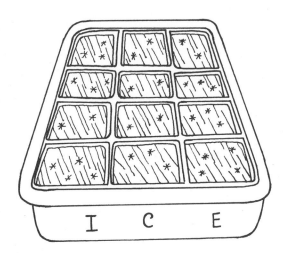

817 SHUT THAT DOOR

In case of a power cut, keep the fridge and freezer doors closed as much as possible. Food should last in the fridge for 4 to 6 hours and in the freezer for 1 to 2 days, depending how full the freezer is – the fuller it is, the longer the food will last.

818 HAVE YOUR CAKE AND FREEZE IT

If you want to freeze a cake or dessert but aren't sure you're going to want the whole lot in one go, why not cut it before freezing. Then you can take out one or two slices at a time, as and when you need them. If buying frozen, though, it's not safe to defrost to cut, then refreeze.

816 HERB CUBES

One of the reasons so many people like shop-bought sauces is that they never have the right ingredients to hand. Stock up with herbs that won't last in the refrigerator, like basil or parsley, by finely chopping and freezing with a small amount of water in ice-cube trays. When you need herbs for a recipe, just toss in a cube.

819 REHEAT YOUR RICE

Freeze leftover cooked long grain or brown rice (other varieties tend to get sticky) for quick use later. Cool the cooked rice before packaging in plastic freezer storage bags and freeze flat. Remember, rice can only be reheated once, so only defrost as much as you need. Also, cooked rice should never be stored at room temperature.

820 BAG THE CUBES

If you're freezing food leftovers or baby meals in ice-cube trays, put the trays in a large plastic bag before you freeze them. This will cut out the air and stop the tops of them from drying out as they freeze, which means they'll keep longer.

821 STORE UP A TV DINNER

Instead of ordering a takeaway when you can't be bothered to cook, make your own 'emergency' TV dinners using leftovers by investing in a three-section reusable plastic container. Fill up each section with protein, vegetable and starch respectively. If all three sections aren't full after one meal, fill up with leftovers from your next meal.

822 BATCH YOUR BROWNING

Browning beef mince (ground beef) can be time consuming, and also messy. Try browning a large batch all in one go when you've got a spare hour or so, then freeze it in your usual-sized portions. Remove it from the freezer and defrost as you need to. Remember not to refreeze it.

823 NO NEED TO CRY

Many people object to chopping onions because it makes them cry. Put a stop to regular tears by preparing 20 or so onions at a time – peel and chop them all, then freeze in a plastic bag. Be aware, though, that they may soften and lose a little of their flavour in freezing.

824 ACCUMULATE A STEW

When you have a spoonful or so of vegetables such as beans, peas or corn left over after a meal, put in a freezer container or bag in the freezer instead of throwing them away. Then, once you've accumulated enough, use your veggie leftovers to make a stew or soup.

825 FLATTEN BAGS

Freeze ground meat in 500 g (1 lb) portions and place in freezer storage bags. Flatten out to the edges of the bag and remove all the air before sealing then freezing. These flat bags of ground meat stack neatly in the freezer, thaw quickly, and it's easy just to break off a bit and reseal.

826 DON'T WASTE WINE

Next time you have a glass or so of wine
left in the bottle that you just can't finish,
don't throw it away. Freeze it in an ice-cube
tray then pop the cubes into a sealed bag
and use in recipes that require a little wine
– and avoid having to open a new
bottle before you need to.

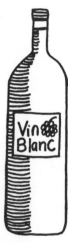
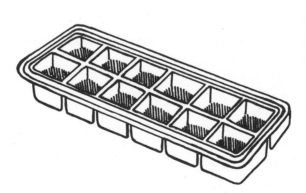

827 GO GINGERLY

Fresh ginger is a great addition to many recipes, but you only need a little and it can be messy to grate. Try freezing it when you buy it then grating as much as you need straight from frozen.

828 KEEP IT TIGHT

The tighter you wrap foods before freezing, the better they will last because fewer ice crystals, which dry the food out, will form. Make sure air is removed from bags and larger items are well wrapped.

829 BULK UP YOUR BACON

Bacon is a great protein-filled snack, but the mess it creates in the kitchen can put people off cooking it. Try buying in bulk, cooking, cooling and then freezing. When you want a snack, you can simply microwave a few rashers.

830 BABY PURÉES

Instead of buying baby food in jars, which may contain preservatives, make up a big batch of puréed vegetables and freeze it in ice cube trays. Defrost one or two ice cubes for each meal.

831 A STRONG BASE

Frozen sauce bases are great for when you don't have time to cook. Try freezing small portions of white sauce that you can defrost, and add cocoa for a chocolate sauce or cheese to make a cheese sauce. You can also freeze a tomato-based sauce.

832 SQUEEZE OUT THE AIR

When you're freezing foods, reducing the amount of air in packages not only helps your freezer to work more efficiently by making packages less bulky, but also prevents ice crystals forming on foods.

meal planning

833 COOK UP A STORM

If you live alone, it can be difficult to muster up the energy to cook a healthy meal for yourself. Try cooking up meals in batches and freezing them, or cook extra and use the leftovers for the next night or two.

834 MAKE GRAFFITI

Don't be afraid to annotate your recipe books when you make changes – instead of using them as food bibles, think of them as starting points and use your own creativity to make healthy changes, making notes as you go. It's usually a good idea to make the original recipe first so that you can compare with any alterations.

835 ONLINE ADVICE

If you're having problems making a meal or menu plan for you or your family, visit one of the increasingly popular menu-planning websites online, some of which even offer weekly menus and shopping lists – so all you have to do is the cooking!

836 ONE-POT COOKING

If you're cooking for one or two, preparing one-dish meals such as beef, barley and vegetable stew, chicken or turkey casserole, vegetarian chilli con carne, or fish and vegetables roasted in a foil package will give you the benefits of home cooking without the hassle.

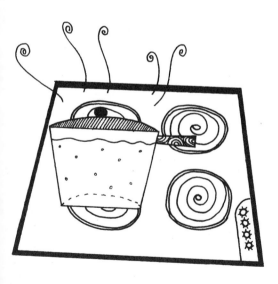

837 TICK THE RIGHT BOXES

To make sure you and your family are getting the right levels of nutrients in your diet, make yourself a weekly or fortnightly meal planner. Include tick boxes for essential nutrients – that way, you can check at a glance whether your diet is balanced and healthy.

838 PLAN YOUR SHOP

Planning your meals for a week or two at a time and then putting together a grocery list with everything you need to cook those meals will cut your trips to the supermarket down to one a week – giving you more time to cook up all those fresh ingredients. You'll be less tempted by fast foods, too.

839 BE AN EARLY BIRD

It might be tempting to lie in for a few extra minutes each morning and skip breakfast, but studies have shown that breakfast eaters are slimmer and perform better at work. Set your alarm five minutes earlier than normal and sit down to eat before you leave the house.

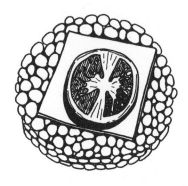

840 MEALY MOUTHED

Redefine a 'meal' – if you're short on time or energy, make a nutritious snack rather than a full meal, but make sure you serve it on a plate rather than eating it on the go. Try healthy snacks such as rice cakes with cheese, olives and tomatoes, or oatcakes with apple and cheese slices.

841 SAVE YOUR PLANS

Keep hold of each week's menu plans, especially when you feel they have worked well, and you will soon be able to start using previous plans for reference, or even repeat successful weeks in their entirety.

842 BE RIGID

A really rigid meal plan and schedule makes the early days of a diet much easier to stick to because it eliminates choice, helping you to deal more easily with temptation. Try to stick to it for at least five days, preferably two weeks, before you get in the swing.

843 NO GOING OFF

Plan your meals around the things that go off most quickly. To avoid soggy veg, for instance, if you buy a big bag of carrots, try to include them in several dinner recipes. Eat them as snacks, too, and use them up by making a carrot cake towards the end of the week.

844 FREE UP FIVE MINUTES

Many people have a problem with meal planning, because they can never find the time. Make a five-minute slot in your day or week to sit down with a cup of tea or cold drink and plan at least your day's, if not your week's, meals. The more you do it, the easier it gets.

845 MEAL FILE

Make yourself a family meal planning file. Keep your previous week's plans in it as well as blank paper for shopping lists, recipes you want to try and any coupons you might have cut out and saved.

846 TEAR OUT A PAGE

Many magazines and newspapers now contain recipes which you may want to try, and these are often aimed at healthy eating. Create a 'healthy eating' recipe folder or scrapbook to keep them all in once place, and use different headings to make the recipes easy to access.

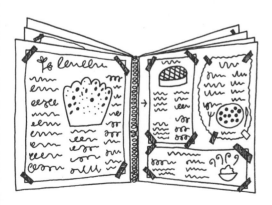

847 CHECK YOUR STORES

Don't forget what's already in your cupboards. Every week or month, look through your kitchen store cupboards to see if there are any foods you can use to plan your meals around. That way, you'll reduce food wastage and give yourself some ideas as well.

848 THINK OF THE FREEZER

Think ahead when planning meals and use your freezer. If you're making something that freezes well like a lasagne or a spaghetti sauce, a stew or casserole, make double and freeze the second portion for those days where you just don't have any time to cook.

849 ADD FRUITY FLAVOUR

Get a vitamin boost by adding fruit to flavour main meals as well as puddings – cook rice in a mixture of water and apple juice, sprinkle broccoli or spinach with raisins, sunflower seeds or chopped almonds, or simmer carrots and parsnips in orange juice.

850 SLIP IN A QUICKIE

Although going to the supermarket once a week is a good way to save time and avoid overspending, it may not always be possible for all items. If you buy a lot of fresh fruit and vegetables you may want to include only half a week's worth of items on your list, and to make a second quick trip during the week for the rest.

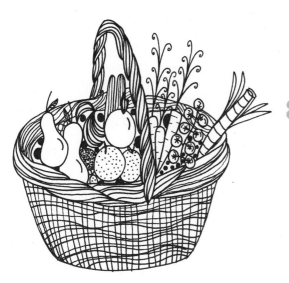

851 BE REALISTIC

When you're planning meals, remember to make allowances for days when you don't have a lot of time. If you know Tuesdays are always stressful, plan something simple for that day like leftover meat and steamed vegetables or salad.

852 BALANCE YOUR INTAKE

Planning meals is a great idea because you can make sure you balance your meals both nutritionally and in terms of cost. If you plan an expensive meal one night, balance it with a pasta dish or a cheaper vegetarian meal the next.

853 IN FULL VIEW

Stick your weekly or bi-weekly menu on your fridge or other prominent place and plan ahead every day. Make a note on your plan if you need to take something out of the freezer, for instance, or if you can prepare part of the meal in advance.

tastes & flavours

854 FRUIT UP YOUR FISH

Don't just stick to serving vegetables with your evening meals – fruit tastes good with fish and meat and is a great way to increase your vitamin and antioxidant intake. Try mango and papaya with tuna, apple with chicken, or pineapple with pork.

855 ADD FLAVOUR LATER

For dishes that take a long time to cook, beware of overflavouring with herbs and spices, which often develop stronger flavour the longer they cook. Add very few herbs and spices at the beginning and an hour before serving add more if you think the dish needs it.

856 DRIED MEANS LESS

Fresh herbs are a great way to get flavour and an added fresh vitamin boost into your dishes, but they're not always available. Remember if you're using dried herbs they're much more pungent than fresh – you need on average one third of the fresh amount.

857 TOAST YOUR SPICES

Whenever possible, grind whole spices in a grinder or mortar and pestle just prior to using. Toasting whole spices in a dry skillet over medium heat before grinding will bring out even more flavour, but be careful not to burn them.

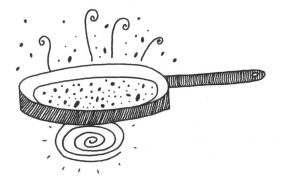

858 OREGANO AND GO

The herb oregano is high in antioxidants, and tastes great finely chopped and scattered over salads, grilled meats and fish. Fresh oregano is also very good added to Italian dishes like pizza, pasta and Bolognese sauces.

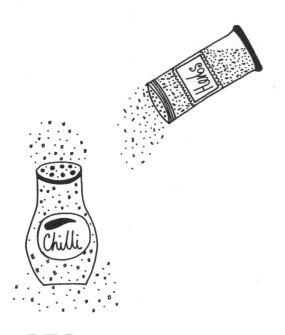

860 STICK WITH STEVIA

Instead of using refined white sugar as a sweetener, go for a natural-sweetening option with the no-calorie herb stevia, a herb from Paraguay with a slightly liquorice aftertaste that is approximately 100 to 400 times sweeter than sugar. It can be purchased in most health food shops and can be used for cooking or baking.

861 MORE CINNAMON LESS SUGAR

In baked spiced recipes like muffins and biscuits, try reducing the amount of sugar in your recipes by half and doubling the cinnamon. Not only will the cinnamon taste help retain sweetness with the least calories possible, it has also been shown to help control blood sugar levels.

859 SHAKE A FLAVOUR FEAST

Add flavour to your food on the plate without using oils and other calorie-filled flavour enhancers by creating your own flavour shakers. Choose your favourite dried herbs and spices and combine in a sugar or salt pot to give flavour without fat – try chilli and chives or basil and oregano.

862 HEALTHIER SWEETNESS

Try natural alternatives to sugar in baking and for sweetening drinks and desserts. Barley malt, rice syrup and granulate cane juice all contain as many calories as sugar, but they also have added minerals and vitamins so are slightly healthier.

863 MUNCH A MACADAMIA

If you love shortbread or buttery biscuits, try closing your eyes and snacking on a handful of macadamia nuts instead. With a rich, buttery taste because of their healthy unsaturated fats, they are filling as well as being low in carbohydrates and high in magnesium, iron and calcium.

864 DON'T CAST AWAY THE CARAWAY

Caraway seeds add a nutty, almost liquorice flavour to foods and are often used in rye breads and other speciality baking. Use them instead of salt to flavour cooked vegetables such as parsnips, carrots and beetroot. They're delicious in parsnip soup and pork and tomato casserole.

865 TREAD GINGERLY

Dried ginger is quite different from fresh. It has a slightly sweet flavour and a hint of citrus as well as the characteristic ginger kick. It can be used to replace sugar in recipes containing fruits like apple and pear, and instead of salt to enhance the flavour of chicken, turkey and rice.

866 MAKE IT WITH MACE

Experiment with spices to replace salt and complement your food. If you find nutmeg too overpowering, try mace. Mace is ground from the covering of the nutmeg seed and is warmer and more delicate in flavour. Use in sauces and meat stews and sprinkled on to vegetables.

867 STAR SUGAR SUBSTITUTE

Instead of piling sugar into your puddings, think of alternatives like star anise and liquorice, which can add a delicious tang without piling on the calories, especially if you combine it with using low-fat yogurt or crème fraiche.

868 GO NATURAL

Replace high-fat sour cream in recipes and as a garnish with low-fat natural yogurt instead. Not only does it contain fewer calories, but if you buy a live version it also contains bacteria which are beneficial to your digestive system. Or substitute half and half if you want to keep the taste but reduce the calories.

869 SPRINKLE SOME SPICE

To easily reduce sugar in sweet recipes without losing out on taste, try substituting spices like cardamom, cinnamon, nutmeg or vanilla, which will enhance the impression of sweetness without adding calories. You can replace the sugar in recipes by between a half and a third without altering the result.

870 CLOVES FOR MEMORY

Cloves are not only great for adding their characteristic flavour, they also contain chemicals which aid digestion. Cloves are also believed to improve mental clarity and memory, so adding them to slow-cooking spiced dishes like stews and curries is a very good idea all round.

871 GARLIC ON A STICK

For the flavour and health benefits of garlic in cooking without actually having to bite through the flesh, stick a whole clove of garlic on a toothpick and add to soups and stews – that way, you'll be able to find and remove it easily before serving.

872 MAKE YOUR OWN MILK

You can make your own healthy low-fat buttermilk for recipes by mixing one cup (235 ml or ½ pint) of plain yogurt with either one teaspoon cream of tartar or one cup of milk and a tablespoon of vinegar.

873 ADD MUSHROOMS TO TASTE

Instead of mayonnaise and creamy dressings, think about ways you can add interest to your salads without adding fat. Raw, chopped or whole mushrooms are a great way to add taste.

quick fixers

874 GET IT RIGHT WITH RICE

If you want a boost of energy in a hurry, which will keep you going for hours until you next eat, try whipping yourself up a simple and healthy carbohydrate treat – mix cooked brown rice with herbs and lemon juice and sprinkle with toasted sunflower or pumpkin seeds.

875 COOK UP AN OMELETTE

If you've only got a few minutes for supper, an omelette with vegetables like spinach, onion and broccoli makes a quick healthy meal. Use lots of vegetables and just enough egg to hold it together, then add salad for an extra health boost.

876 A QUICK FIX

For a quick, nutritious TV dinner, bake or microwave a sweet potato and instead of butter, drizzle with a little honey or maple syrup and sprinkle with cinnamon and/or nutmeg. Then serve with salad and a protein source such as fish or meat. Kids love it, too.

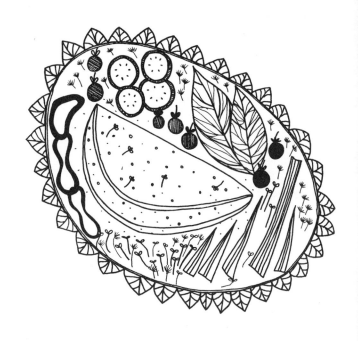

877 TASTE THE TABOULLEH

For a fresh and healthy alternative to pasta or rice, make up a bowl of Lebanese tabouIIeh, which is made from cracked wheat and traditionally contains large amounts of healthy parsley as well as tomato, onion and extra virgin olive oil.

878 GLAZED FRUIT DESSERT

Cook yourself a decadent dessert that's a lot healthier than it might seem by glazing pineapple with rum or brandy and frying or grilling until warm. Serve with a sauce made from reduced orange juice, cinnamon and nutmeg and a spoonful of natural yogurt.

879 GET SAUCY

Make your own light pasta sauce using fat-free or low-fat cottage cheese puréed or whisked together with a touch of evaporated skimmed milk, lemon juice and a little rosemary. Shred some spinach into the dish just before serving for colour and an added health boost.

880 BIND WITH BEANS

Instead of creamy dips, use the binding power of beans to knock up healthy eastern-style hors-d'oeuvres. Purée kidney beans with garlic, red chilli, powdered cumin seed, lime juice, olive oil and tomatoes, then stir in chopped onion and coriander leaves.

881 A HEALTHY BLEND

To make a healthy breakfast smoothie, blend strawberries and papaya (low-GI foods with a high antioxidant content) and half a banana (for blood sugar regulation) with skimmed milk (for calcium) ice cubes and a squeeze of maple syrup (for taste!).

882 BAKE A WHOLESOME TREAT

Bake up a batch of healthy muffins for family breakfasts and snacks. If you make your own you can include only the best ingredients – and you'll know they won't contain preservatives and artificial flavourings or colourings. Choose ingredients like oats, banana, honey, raisins, bran and blueberries.

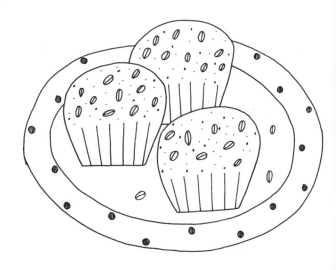

883 START THE DAY WELL

For a great carb-free breakfast, have a bowl of yogurt – which has digestive benefits as well as calcium – and fresh berries for a morning vitamin boost. Add some flaxseed oil or ground flaxseeds for a dose of omega-3 oils for a perfect start.

884 BOOST BREAKFAST ENERGY

Don't only use fruit for your morning smoothie. Kick start the day with an energy-giving blend of green tea (for a healthy caffeine boost), carrot juice (for carbohydrates) and your chosen fruit (try mango and banana or apricots and plums). Add low-fat natural yogurt as a filler.

885 HOME IS BEST

Make sure you eat breakfast at home rather than on the go, as take-away breakfasts are often laden with calories and sugar. A regular latte with a flapjack adds up to an astounding 750 calories, compared with around 250 for a bowl of cereal and a cup of tea or coffee with skimmed milk.

886 GRILLED FRUIT

For a quick, healthy pudding, try making fruit kebabs. Peel and chop fruit into similar sizes, then alternate on a skewer and grill for a few minutes on each side. Serve alone or with natural yogurt and a dash of honey or maple syrup.

887 TAKE A CHEESY DIP

Instead of dipping crudités and raw vegetables into dips like taramasalata and sour cream, which can be fattening, make your own healthy version using cottage cheese, spring onions and garlic.

888 BREAKFAST ON MUESLI

Set yourself up for the day with a bowl of museli with low-fat milk, fruit and low-fat yogurt. The oats and wholegrains will help you to feel full until lunchtime.

889 BUTTER AN APPLE

Cut one apple into thin slices and top with 1–2 tbsp of peanut butter. Include a glass of milk or a small carton of low-fat yogurt for an unusual, all-round healthy breakfast.

880 NOT MUSH-ROOM FOR MEAT

Mushrooms have a great meaty texture and are an easy and cheap way to cut down your meat intake. Choose grilled portabello mushrooms in place of a burger (or in place of the bun if you're cutting out bread).

881 COOK WHEN YOU RISE

Don't be afraid to use your oven in the morning. Eggs with wholemeal bread are a great way to start the day, giving you a good measure of protein and carbohydrate. Add a piece of fresh fruit for total balance.

882 PICK THE RIGHT PASTA

Substitute wholewheat pasta for plain pasta in recipes, particularly in the evening when you don't want a quick release of sugar into your system.

883 GET THE GREEN BENEFITS

Instead of iceberg lettuce in your salad, which has fairly low levels of nutrients (but is still better than no salad) choose leafier, darker greens like chicory, kale, rocket or watercress, which contain higher levels of nutrients.

894 BULK UP WITH VEG

If you're making a meat stew or casserole, halve the amount of meat required and substitute it with vegetables. That way, you'll cut the calories and give yourself a bit of added vegetable goodness, not to mention reducing the costs.

895 DITCH THE GRANOLA

Granola might seem like a healthy breakfast choice because it's packed with fruit and carbohydrates, but unfortunately it's also full of fat and sugar, and is one of the most calorific cereals on the market. Stick to low-fat muesli instead, or dilute it with some healthy oats or bran. It's also delicious used as a topping for low-fat yogurt.

896 SKIM OFF SOME WEIGHT

Skimmed milk contains about half the calories of whole milk (80 compared to about 150 for one cup), and semi-skimmed milk sits somewhere in between. Lower-fat versions also provide the body with more calcium, so they're the healthier choice, unless you're underweight or a child.

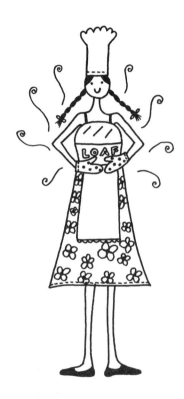

897 BAKE YOUR OWN BREAD

Bread is often full of additives such as palm oil and even hormones, so one of the best ideas for family cooking is to invest in a breadmaking machine. They're relatively cheap and very easy to use – and you'll know exactly what your kids are eating.

898 LOVE YOUR LENTILS

Serve brown or wild rice or lentils instead of white rice as a filler with your meals. The rice doesn't taste very different and because you're choosing wholegrains they're better for your digestive system and have a lower GI.

healthy preparation

899 UP-TEMPO EGGS

When you're going to beat egg whites for a recipe, let the eggs sit at room temperature for 30 minutes before using them. The egg whites will then beat to a greater volume.

900 CHOOSE QUALITY INGREDIENTS

Choosing quality, rather than quantity, when it comes to cooking can help you stay healthy because you'll get a great deal of flavour without having to pile up your plate. Try a dash of balsamic vinegar for dressings or truffle oil instead of butter in mashed potato.

901 TAKE A WORLD VIEW

Think global and try incorporating the healthiest part of other cultures' eating habits into your diet – the olive oil and fresh vegetables of the Mediterranean, Japan's variety of small, tasty portions, the fish of Scandinavia, and Latin America's fibre-filled wholegrains.

902 BE A FRESH PHYT-ER

Adding a variety of fresh herbs to cooking is a great idea because each herb contains different types and levels of health-giving phytochemicals, which are used in the body to help mop up free radicals and fight damage. Add them freshly picked just before serving for the best effect.

903 RUN THE COARSE

It's healthier to use coarse ground salt than powdered varieties in measured recipes. This is because the lower surface area to volume ratio means the food absorbs less of the potentially damaging sodium.

904 SKIM OFF THE CALORIES

Preparing your desserts with skimmed milk instead of whole milk will save around 63 calories and 8 g of fat per serving, so use skimmed milk whenever you can, and use single (light) cream instead of double (heavy) where possible, too.

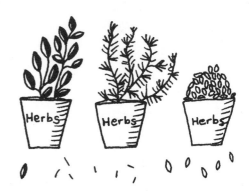

905 BASE IT ON STOCK

If you want to marinade but don't want your fish or meat swimming in oil, use fruit juice or stock to form the base instead. You'll still help the meat retain flavour and tenderness without using extra oil.

906 USE DRY MARINADES

Instead of marinating meats in oil and your favourite spices, rub the dried spices into the meat instead. That way, you won't be adding any extra fat to the meat and you'll get the same yummy taste.

907 LET IT EXPAND

To ensure the optimum taste of meat, allow it to come to room temperature for half an hour to an hour before cooking. This will allow the meat to expand, helping the taste to spread evenly during cooking.

908 MEASURE THE OIL

Don't splash oil into the pan before frying or stir-frying without measuring it – you might use more than you need. Most frying only needs a teaspoon or less of oil per serving.

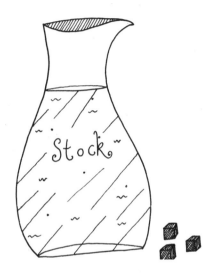

908 SPLIT YOUR EGGS

To help your low-fat diet, separate out the yolks and whites of your eggs so that you only use the more calorific yolks if you really need them. Do this by breaking the egg in half then transferring the yolk from one side of the shell to the other, while collecting the white that falls out in a bowl below.

910 HOW TO CHOP ONIONS

To chop onions the easy way, start by cutting off the stem end, then peel the skin back to the root, but keep it attached. Holding the skin to steady the onion, cut towards the root end but not through the root, then slice finely across the onion from the stem end.

911 BAG THE DRESSING

To limit the amount of oily dressing you use on salads, don't pour it directly on to the salad in a bowl. Instead, start by putting all your salad ingredients into ziplock bag. Add a small amount of salad dressing and shake the bag before dividing into individual bowls.

912 OAT ROLLING

Rolled oats are quicker to cook but not quite as good for you as unrolled oats, which have a very low GI rating (meaning they release energy very slowly). If you want the best of both worlds, blitz your unrolled oats in the blender to turn them into instant oatmeal!

913 MIX IN SOME OIL

If your recipe requires eggs but you don't want the calories of egg yolk, use the egg white mixed with a teaspoon of olive oil instead. This gives a better consistency than using the whites on their own, which can make the mixture too light, plus extra health benefits.

914 THE WHOLE STORY

Whenever possible, avoid buying salad leaves in ready-prepared bags available in supermarkets, as they have often been washed with chlorine products to kill bugs. Buy lettuces whole instead, and wash them yourself.

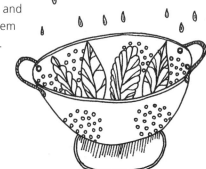

915 AN OATY COAT

Use rolled oats or crushed bran cereal instead of breadcrumbs on your fish fillets or chicken drumsticks – you'll use less because it's more powdery and it will give you a wholegrain boost into the bargain!

916 FLOUR YOUR RECIPES

Instead of using egg as a thickener in recipes, use a tablespoon of wholewheat flour, which will play the same thickening role but with far fewer calories. If the egg is being used as a binding agent, use flour and oil instead.

917 DITCH THE SALT

Unsalted butter can be substituted for normal salted butter in most recipes. You won't usually notice any difference in taste, but you will be cutting down on salt.

918 MAKE DO WITHOUT MAYO

Instead of mayonnaise, combine low-fat yogurt with low-fat cottage cheese and mix well together. If you like, you can add extra flavour with a little mustard, garlic or some fresh or dried herbs.

919 STUFF A MUSHROOM

Instead of filling your poultry with a stuffing that's heavy on breadcrumbs, substitute half the breadcrumbs for chopped mushrooms. They'll keep their form, taste really good and cut down your carbohydrate intake.

920 BAN THE BOOZE

Alcohol is an optional ingredient in many recipes like stews and pasta sauces and gives a distinctive flavour. If you'd prefer a lower-calorie option, you can substitute with stock in most savoury dishes, and fruit juice in most sweet recipes.

921 KEEP IT LEMON FRESH

When preparing ripe avocados, to avoid the flesh turning brown and looking unattractive when exposed to air, immediately place the cut fruit (flesh side down) in lemon juice until ready for use. Covering the cut surface tightly with clingfilm (plastic wrap) and putting it in the fridge will also stop it changing colour. Use within a couple of days.

equipment & utensils

922 RACK UP YOUR HEALTH

Invest in a roasting rack for your Sunday dinners. The principle is that the rack elevates the meat or poultry, allowing fat to drip into the pan below and reducing the amount of fat on the roast. A rack is also a good idea for cooking sausages and chicken pieces in the oven.

923 PUT A LID ON IT

If you're stir-frying, invest in a lid for your frying pan or wok. Covering will increase the humidity of your cooking, meaning you can use less oil to achieve non-stick results.

924 BUY QUALITY

Invest in a set of quality non-stick pots and pans so you can bake and sauté without adding extra oil. If you can only afford one or two, go for a frying pan first, then a large pan for pasta, and so on.

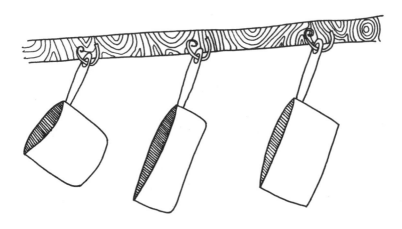

925 ACHIEVE GRATE THINGS

Instead of relying on slices of cheese, use a cheese grater, which will help you use smaller portions because it adds air to the cheese. Your grater should also have a thin slicer with which you can cut thinner slices than you would by hand.

926 MAKE THE CUT

Invest in one good quality kitchen knife rather than an array of cheaper ones, and keep it sharp. It will help with healthy eating by allowing you to cut nearer to the skin of fruit and vegetables, where more nutrients are stored, and to cut the fat off meat without wasting the flesh.

927 GET A GRILL

To cook your food more healthily, especially if you rely on fried foods, consider investing in one of the many varieties of fat-free electric grills on the market, or a simple griddle (grill) pan There's no need to add any oil to these – just get the pan nice and hot and cook as you would do when pan frying.

cooking & serving

928 STICK TO THE SKINS

Next time you plan on serving mashed potatoes, just stop for a minute and consider that the act of mashing will raise their glycaemic index as well as causing loss of healthy vitamins. Serving them baked in their skins with a low-fat filling such as cottage cheese is much healthier.

929 ROAST POTATOES

Instead of using your deep-fat fryer to make chips (French fries), create a healthy version by roasting thick slices of sweet potato in olive oil – leave the skins on for added goodness.

930 A CAKEY COOKIE

If you're making biscuits or cookies, choose the soft drop, more cakey version rather than the rolled variety – they generally contain more air per serving and therefore fewer calories.

931 ADVICE OF A MEDIUM

One of the main benefits of eating fish and meat is the essential amino acids they provide, which help the body with energy and the growth and repair of cells. Moderate cooking enhances this benefit, but overcooking can kill them off, so choose medium-cooked meat and fish.

932 ADJUST TIMINGS

It's important to cook grains for long enough for the body to absorb their nutrients, but be aware that cooking times aren't set in stone. Grains that have been in storage for a long time will take longer to cook through than recently harvested ones, and toasted grains often cook faster because the breakdown process has already begun.

933 BUY PRE-SOAKED

It can be difficult to add wholegrains to recipes because of the soaking or cooking time required. Many supermarkets now sell pre-soaked varieties which cook in 30–45 minutes, or try cooking up a batch at once and keeping it (for 2–3 days in the fridge or several months in the freezer).

934 WOBBLE YOUR FRUIT

Instead of fattening puddings, why not serve fruit set in jelly? It's a favourite with adults and children alike and looks smart and sleek served in individual portions, with the added bonus of being very low in calories. Use apple juice instead of sugar to sweeten.

935 COOK UP A JUS

Instead of serving your roast meals with traditional thick gravy, which can add calories to a meal because of the flour and fat it contains, try a small amount of meat juices. Add a dash of lemon juice or white wine for poultry and a little red wine or balsamic vinegar for red meats.

936 OIL QUALITY TEST

Test the quality of your olive oil by frying a few drops in a pan – really good quality oil which has the most health benefits will stay green and light. If it turns dark and loses its shine, it's not a good quality oil.

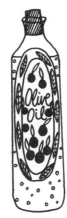

937 BRAISE THE FLAVOUR

One of the healthiest ways of cooking meat, particularly tougher cuts which need longer, is braising. This method involves browning in a pan, then slowly cooking with a small quantity of liquid such as water or stock, to retain tenderness without adding fat.

938 DOUBLE YOUR DISH

If you're preparing a family meal such as shepherd's pie, beef stew or lasagne, make double and freeze half of it so you've got a healthy emergency family meal to hand if you ever need it.

939 COOK THINGS SLOWLY

If you're busy all day and don't have the time or energy to cook a healthy meal when you get home every night, think about investing in a slow cooker or slow steamer. You'll have a healthy meal to come home to – and you're less likely to think about snacking when you get back.

940 FLAKE YOUR FISH

For added crunch with fewer calories, use cornflakes instead of breadcrumbs to coat fish fillets. Not only do cornflakes contain fewer calories than breadcrumbs, they are less absorbent and give a lighter covering, so will absorb less oil.

941 SQUASH WINTER BLUES

Butternut squash is a fantastic winter food which keeps its healthy nutrients and betacarotene for months, but it can be hard to cut and prepare. Prick a few holes and put it into the microwave oven on high power for 1 minute, then let it sit for a minute and it should be easier to cut. Now there's no excuse!

942 AFTERNOON ZEST

Citrus fruits are a great way of getting a vitamin boost and their aromas are thought to help boost energy and alertness, so they're a great afternoon pick-me-up. The zest is great sprinkled on yogurts for pudding – grate and store the rinds of your oranges, lemons or grapefruits instead of throwing away.

943 TOWEL AWAY GREASE

When grease settles on broth or soup, float a piece of paper towel lightly on top of the liquid and it will absorb grease. Don't allow it to become sodden – you may have to use more than one piece – and lightly lift to remove excess oil.

944 LET MEAT STAND

After cooking a joint of meat, you should always let it stand for 10–15 minutes (depending on the size of the joint) to 'rest'. The meat will actually continue to gently cook during this time, which allows the juices to permeate the meat and makes it taste more full and tender.

945 LETTUCE ON STAND-BY

If you don't like washing your salad leaves every time you prepare a salad or garnish, keep a ready-washed store in your fridge. Wash and dry whole lettuce leaves (breaking them up causes them to go limp quickly) and dry carefully with kitchen towel (being careful not to squash them), then store in a large plastic bag in the fridge.

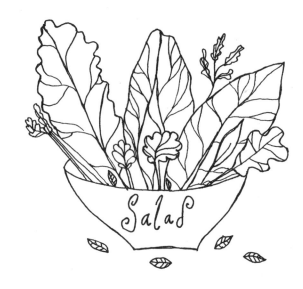

946 RINSE YOUR MINCE

When making meals using beef mince (ground beef) at home, try this fat-reducing tip: put the browned mince into a strainer and rinse with hot water until the water runs clear, removing the fat in the process.

947 REDUCE YOUR OIL

Use your microwave to cook foods without covering them in oil. Microwave cooking relies on water content, not fat, so is often lower in calories than oven-cooked food. It's especially useful for fish and vegetables.

948 MASH WITH WATER

Save on fat when making mashed potatoes by setting aside some of the water the potatoes were cooked in and adding it to the potatoes when mashing them. The potatoes will be just as fluffy without butter.

949 USE A VINEGAR SHIELD

If you're making a pasta salad, cut down the amount of dressing or mayonnaise your pasta soaks up by tossing it in a little vinegar first, to coat it with a fat-repelling layer.

950 TOSS IN HOT WATER

Instead of tossing your cooked pasta with oil to prevent it sticking, use stock instead, or a little hot water. That way, you won't be adding any extra calories to your meal, and you can enjoy a little more sauce instead!

951 ALL BY ITSELF

Balsamic vinegar makes a great fat-free salad dressing. Try it sprinkled on ripe tomatoes with some fresh basil on top. For extra taste try the really thick varieties – they're expensive but you only need a few drops.

952 SKIM OFF THE FAT

For a low-fat soup, the best way to remove all the excess fat is to cool then refrigerate the soup. Then simply skim off the hardened fat when it's cold.

953 USE A LEAF TO CUT FAT

If you're making a quick soup and you want to get rid of the fat from the top, but haven't got time to refrigerate it, try throwing in a large lettuce leaf. The fat will stick to it, then you can remove and discard it.

954 NON-BISCUIT BASE

If your recipe calls for biscuits, such as crushed digestives (graham crackers) for the base of a cheesecake, try crushed no-sugar-added oatcakes instead. They're a healthy alternative, made from wholegrains and full of fibre and vitamin B. Muesli is another good alternative.

955 CUT THE ICE

Ice cubes are another great soup or casserole de-greaser. Simply drop in a few ice cubes and watch the fat and grease cling to them, then remove (before they have time to melt) and throw away. Or wrap them in muslin and drag over the surface instead.

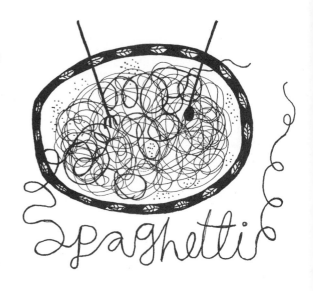

956 DITCH THE ALCOHOL

Contrary to popular belief, alcohol in recipes doesn't burn off entirely with cooking. Even after an hour, 25% of the alcohol can remain, and three hours later there is still a residue of 5%. Choose alternatives like dealcoholized wine, vinegar or fruit juices instead.

957 NON-STICK SPAGHETTI

To make sure you don't pile your plate too high with spaghetti, stop it sticking together (especially if you're using fresh rather than dried pasta) by washing off the starch with boiling water once it's cooked. The sauce won't cling as well, but you'll be able to better control portion sizes.

958 SOAK UP FAT

Place a few pieces of dry bread in the grill (broiler) pan when grilling meats to soak up dripping fat. This not only means your meats will be leaner, it eliminates smoking fat and therefore reduces fire risk.

959 JUICE YOUR MASH

It might not sound a likely combination, but try squeezing some fresh lemon juice into your mashed potatoes instead of butter or oil. Season with freshly ground black pepper for a no-added-fat mash that is flavourful and goes fantastically well with roast chicken.

960 DON'T OVERCOOK FISH

Fish tastes best when it's cooked just enough, and not overcooked. As a general rule, cook for 4–5 minutes each side for every inch of thickness. When it's done, the flesh should just start to separate into flakes when tested with a fork, and should appear opaque throughout. Some fish, such as tuna and salmon, can be served medium rare.

961 SAUTÉ IN WINE

Instead of sautéeing in butter or oil, use wine, especially if you have some handy ice cubes of leftover wine in the freezer. Otherwise, a quick splosh and you'll have a low-calorie sautéed meal.

outdoor entertaining

962 COOL OFF

For picnics, freeze juice or cordial in small plastic water bottles and use them to keep your other food cool and fresh. When they defrost, you'll have a cold drink.

963 THE TWO-HOUR RULE

If you're planning to have take-away foods such as fried chicken or barbecued beef on a picnic, eat them within two hours of pick-up or buy them ahead of time and chill completely before packing the foods into a cooler.

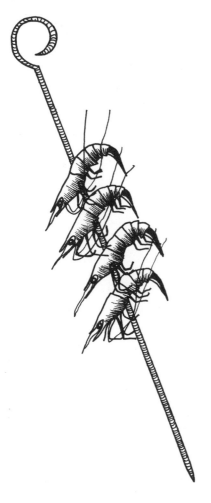

964 SKEW GOOD

Using skewers on the barbecue serves two great roles – first, it allows you to exercise good portion control by making a 'meal on a stick' using vegetables as well as meat or fish. And second, using metal skewers heats up the centre of food, helping it to cook more thoroughly.

965 PACK FOOD TOP DOWN

To help your food stay fresh and cool in the great outdoors, pack foods in the cooler in the order opposite to that which you'll be using them. In other words, pack the food you'll need last at the bottom so it stays cooler longer.

966 KEEP UTENSILS APART

Make sure if you're barbecuing you keep separate utensils for raw and uncooked meat. Using the same tongs to put raw sausages onto the grill and to take cooked ones off could spread harmful bacteria. If you've only got one set of tongs, sterilize them by plunging them into the coals or flames between use.

967 DON'T RE-USE MARINADES

To keep bacteria at bay, never reuse marinades that have come into contact with raw meat, chicken or fish. And don't put the cooked food back into an unwashed container or dish which has been in contact with the marinade.

968 A CLEAN PLATE

When taking foods off the barbecue, put them on a clean plate and not on the same platter that held any raw meat.

969 SEPARATE FOOD AND DRINK

If you're picnicking or eating outdoors, take separate coolers for food and drinks. The drinks cooler will be opened much more often, meaning your food can remain closed and retain its cool air as long as possible.

970 LAST-MINUTE COOLNESS

When preparing chicken, egg, cold meat salads or any recipes featuring mayonnaise, refrigerate as soon as possible and keep cold right up until packing time to ensure they are extra cold.

971 COOLER TO KEEP HOT

Don't forget that cool bags and boxes can be used to keep hot food hot as well as cold food cold. Line the cooler with tea towels (dish towels) for extra insulation and wrap foods well before putting them in and they could stay warm for hours, especially if tightly packed.

972 COOL THINGS DOWN

If you're taking pre-cooked food to eat out at a picnic or barbecue, make sure you make it the night or morning before, so it's got plenty of time to cool right down in the fridge before transportation. Never precook meat and poultry partially before transporting. It must be cooked until done and chilled thoroughly.

973 FREEZE GRAPES

If you want to keep your wine cool in the glass for drinking on hot summer days, use frozen grapes instead of ice cubes. They'll keep the drink cold and they won't dilute it or change the taste as they thaw. Make sure you wash them before freezing.

974 GRILL UP SOME HEALTH

Barbecues don't have to be unhealthy.
Simply choose more of the healthier
foods like chicken, peppers,
aubergines (eggplant),
fish and bananas and
less of the high-fat
sausages, burgers and
marshmallows.

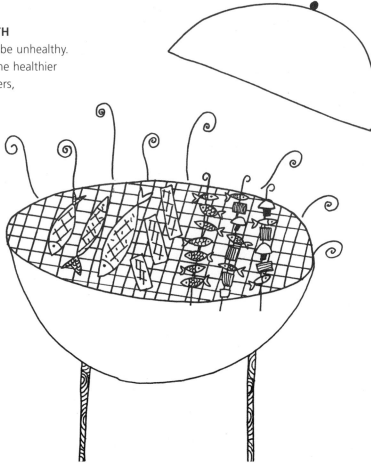

975 GIVE SNACKS THE BOOT

If you've stocked up on treats for a special occasion but are worried you won't be able to resist opening them and tucking in beforehand, use your car as a store. You'll be much less likely to snack if you have to go out to your car to get a treat!

976 MAKE YOUR OWN DIP

Instead of buying fatty dips for your vegetables or crisps, make your own homemade healthy dip with low-fat natural yogurt, lemon juice, garlic and diced cucumber – delicious for summer parties.

hygiene & safety

977 SEPARATE FOOD TYPES

When shopping, keep raw foods away from pre-cooked items. Raw meat and fish are often wrapped but, particularly if they've been bought from a butcher or fishmonger, there's a possibility the outside of bags may also contain bacteria, so separation is safest.

978 WRAP UP FISH

To keep fish fresh, securely wrap it in a plastic bag or moisture-proof paper and store in your refrigerator. You should always use fresh fish within two days, and preferably on the day of purchase. Store frozen seafood for no more than six months.

979 WASH HANDS THOROUGHLY

You know you should wash your hands after handling raw fish and meat but make sure you wash them properly – studies have shown that many people neglect thumbs and the areas between the fingers, as well as the backs of hands. Check the soap has covered the whole area before rinsing with hot water (warm for children).

980 NOW WASH EVERYTHING ELSE

Fresh raw fish can contain bacteria and microbes which can cause illness if ingested without being sterilized by cooking. Make sure you wash hands, cutting boards and utensils after coming into contact with fish.

981 WASH BOTTLES

If you re-use water bottles, make sure you wash them with warm soapy water or put them through the dishwasher from time to time. Although water is clean, it does contain some microbes and you don't want bacteria to build up. You should also wash water-filter jugs between uses.

982 EGG TEST

Lower uncooked eggs into a bowl of water to see if they're past their best. A very fresh egg will immediately sink to the bottom and lie flat on its side. This is because the air cell within the egg is very small. If it settles vertically, it's just about OK, but if it rises to the top, throw it away.

983 THAW RUN-OFF

When meat thaws, lots of liquid can come out of it. This liquid will spread bacteria to any food, plates or surfaces it comes into contact with. Either keep thawing meat in a sealed container at the bottom of the fridge or carefully dispose of the juices and wash your hands.

984 EXTRA CARE

Pregnant women, children and older people are less likely to be able to recover from food poisoning, so they should avoid products which may contain harmful bacteria. Avoid dishes made with raw or undercooked eggs, unpasteurised diary products and soft cheeses, and reheat cook-chill dishes until piping hot.

985 DON'T REPEAT THE REHEAT

If you defrost raw meat and then cook it thoroughly, you can freeze it again, but remember you should never reheat foods more than once. If you want to use a bulky sauce like Bolognese for several meals, reheat individual portions as and when you need them rather than the whole pot.

986 DON'T BE A TECHY

Some believe that hi-tech antimicrobial cutting boards in the kitchen could leach toxins into foods, particularly those that are absorbent like meat, fish and dairy products. Choose wood, marble or steel for safety and durability.

987 A RAW DEAL FOR BOARDS

Try and keep one of the cutting boards in your kitchen for raw meat and fish only. Many people choose plastic versions but there is evidence to show that wood is actually the best choice because of its natural antimicrobial properties.

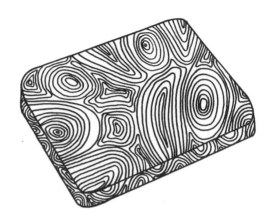

988 GET OFF YOUR METAL

Don't store food in tin or aluminium cans in the fridge or cupboard as the air can cause metal ions to spread into food (unless they are designed for repeated use, such as with golden syrup). If you only want to use half a can, empty the rest into a bowl or other food container and dispose of or recycle the can straight away.

989 YOUR TUM LIKES IT HOT

When you purchase a hot take-away, eat with 2 hours to prevent harmful bacteria from multiplying. If you are not eating within 2 hours, keep your food in the oven set at a high enough temperature to keep the food at or above 60°C (140°F). Check with a food thermometer.

990 THE DANGER ZONE

Harmful bacteria can grow rapidly in food if it's kept in the danger zone (4–60°C/40–140°F), so remember the 2-hour rule and discard any perishable foods left in the danger zone longer than 2 hours.

991 BEAT THE BULGE

If any of your cans start to bulge, throw them away immediately without opening as they could contain nasty bacteria – including the potentially deadly botulism organism which could cause serious harm.

992 DON'T FOIL YOUR ACID

Aluminium kitchen foil can be useful for wrapping and covering foods, but it's best to avoid it for foods that are highly acidic, such as tomatoes, rhubarb, cabbage and soft fruits, because aluminium can affect their taste.

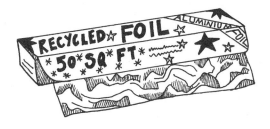

993 CLEAN UP

Remember that housework can burn up to 300 calories an hour, so keeping your kitchen surfaces clean could not only help you prevent food poisoning, it could also help you drop those extra inches! Remember to clean door handles, where bacteria can accumulate.

994 SEARCH FOR THE STEAM

Make sure you always reheat pre-cooked meats until they're steaming hot, which will kill off any bacteria that may cause health problems. You should never eat meat that's only been reheated to lukewarm.

995 FIRE SAFETY

Outfit your kitchen with a fire extinguisher and teach everyone in the family how to use it, even children. Many house fires could be prevented if kitchens were prepared.

996 THROW IT OUT

If you have leftovers from a picnic, only keep them if there is still ice in the cooler and they haven't been out in the sun for too long. There's one basic rule for leftovers – if in doubt, throw it out!

997 DON'T FAN THE FLAMES

If one of your saucepans catches fire, use the lid of the pan to cover the flames and suffocate the fire. Then give the pan a chance to cool down before you move it as movement may cause it to re-ignite.

998 PUT IT OUT WITH SODA

Humble baking soda is the best defence against small kitchen fires – simply throw baking soda at the base of the flames. But don't use this method if the fire is caused by fat or grease, as splashing could result in severe burns.

999 MEASURE FOOD TEMPERATURE

To make your barbecues extra safe, invest in a food thermometer. Burgers, ribs and sausages should be at least 70°C/160°F and poultry 80°C/180°F before you can be sure all the bacteria are killed.

1000 GO FREE RANGE

If you're using raw eggs in a recipe, such as chocolate mousse or mayonnaise, use free-range eggs. Almost no salmonella has been found in free-range eggs.

1001 KEEP THEM APART

Use separate knives and other utensils for raw and cooked meat, so you don't transfer any bacteria to the cooked items. Also, if you are cooking for vegetarians remember to keep any utensils used for any meat product – cooked or raw – away from the vegetables or other ingredients that will be combined.

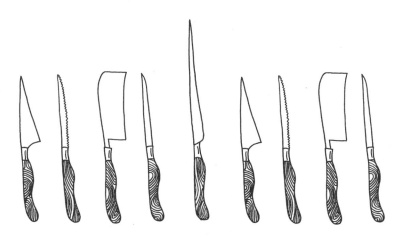

ACKNOWLEDGEMENTS

The author would like to thank Pauline Floyd and Kevin Hall.